PLANET
OBESITY

GARRY EGGER & BOYD SWINBURN

PLANET OBESITY

HOW WE'RE EATING OURSELVES AND THE PLANET TO DEATH

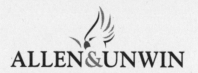

ALLEN&UNWIN

First published in 2010

Allen & Unwin
83 Alexander Street
Crows Nest NSW 2065
Australia
Phone: (61 2) 8425 0100
Fax: (61 2) 9906 2218
Email: info@allenandunwin.com
Web: www.allenandunwin.com

Cataloguing-in-Publication details are available
from the National Library of Australia
www.librariesaustralia.nla.gov.au

ISBN 978 1 74237 362 1

Internal design by Mathematics
Typeset in 10.5/15.5pt Sabon Roman by Post Pre-Press Group, Brisbane
Printed and bound in Australia by McPherson's Printing Group

10 9 8 7 6 5 4 3 2 1

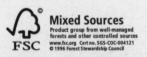

Mixed Sources
Product group from well-managed
forests and other controlled sources
www.fsc.org Cert no. SGS-COC-004121
© 1996 Forest Stewardship Council

CONTENTS

TO BEGIN...   1

1   Hitting The Sweet Spot   3

2   Obesity: Its Part in Our Downfall   10

3   Good Fat versus Bad Fat   19

4   The Role of Inflammation   28

5   Health, 'Illth', Economic Growth and the Sweet Spot   41

6   Linking Obesity, Chronic Disease and the Environment   52

7   The Perfect Storm and the Sour Spot   65

8   Health Promotion for Economists   71

9   Making Corrections   84

10   Just Help Yourself   94

Postscript   107

Notes   111

Acknowledgments   125

Index   127

FIGURES

2.1   An ecological model of obesity   18

3.1   Links between fat and health   26

4.1   The effects of lifestyle on chronic disease   38

6.1   The link between obesity and greenhouse gases   54

6.2   The causes of inflammation   60

10.1   Energy volume and body weight   103

TABLES

4.1   The effects of lifestyle on chronic disease   33

9.1   Global warming potential of gases
        released from combustion of fuels   87

9.2   Potential effects of personal carbon trading
        on individual health and the broader
        environment   91

To our families,
who have been long suffering as a result of
our desire to rid the world of all known problems.

TO BEGIN . . .

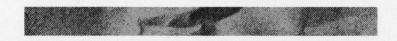

As any sportsman or woman can tell you, there are sweet spots in life, when circumstances come together to create seemingly ideal points in time. Depending on the experience, the participant and the circumstance, these can last for milliseconds—like the sweet strike of a golf club on ball—hours, days, years, or even centuries—like the Roman Empire. For sweet spots apply to populations just as they do to individuals. However, humans have a tendency to overshoot sweet spots by trying to *maximise*, rather than *optimise* the experience. Like Cinderella, we often stay too long at the ball.

In the first part of this book we consider three related worldwide sweet spots that may have already been overshot:

1. Economic growth, which appears to have surpassed its sweet spot, at least in advanced industrialised countries, leading to diminishing returns in human wellbeing and the environment

2. Population levels of body fatness, which, within a range, are optimal for good health, but when pushed by over-consumption can cause obesity and chronic diseases

3. Greenhouse gas emissions, which have increased to the extent that the world's 'sinks' that soak them up are no longer in balance with the sources that create them, leading to environmental disturbances such as climate change.

These three phenomena are not just coincidental, but are causally related, with economic growth, beyond its sweet spot, being the main force pushing both obesity and climate change beyond their respective sweet spots.

Our objective in this book is to create an awareness of these linked and pressing problems of modern life. Solving these problems will be the responsibility of a range of different experts, such as economists, administrators, ecologists, politicians and health scientists—*we* do not pretend to have all the answers. However, in the second part of the book we put forward some suggestions for preventing this confluence of potentially overshot sweet spots from turning decidedly sour. We include a number of 'stealth' interventions, at both the individual and the public health level as we believe they have the potential to help *optimise* our economic, consumption and environmental sweet spots, and pull us back from the path of diminishing returns our desire to *maximise* our experience has led us down.

For make no mistake, overshooting these sweet spots will have serious, potentially catastrophic consequences for the worldwide population. We need to act *now* to keep ourselves and our environment healthy and happy in both the short- and long-term future.

CHAPTER 1

HITTING THE SWEET SPOT

'Any intelligent fool can make things bigger, more complex and more violent. It takes a touch of genius—and a lot of courage—to move in the opposite direction'

ALBERT EINSTEIN

We have a friend who drinks one 350 ml glass of home brew, one 200 ml glass of wine and one 50 ml shot of Scotch a night. Not a millilitre more; not a millilitre less. He always does this after 6 p.m. and before 9 p.m. Ask him why and he'll tell you that it's taken him twenty years, but he now knows that this mix, in those amounts, at that time, enables him to hit his sweet spot every night. Any more and he gets tired and irritable; any less and he doesn't as effectively reduce his workday stress.

In the wider world, the Roman Empire existed for around 800 years, much of which was spent on the rise, and much, as has been famously written, in fall. It's debatable at just which point, and for how long, it achieved its sweet spot. But the time of Hadrian, around 120AD, when the Empire spanned three continents with an army of some 150,000 and a population of around 10 million, was probably close to it.

Similarly, for Winston Churchill and the British Empire, their 'finest hour', arguably followed the defeat of Nazism, while holding Empire in far-flung places, such that the sun never set on some aspect of English influence.

So life fluctuates between good and bad. At the good end there are sweet spots—times, however fleeting, when everything seems just right. (There are also sour spots at the bad end—but we'll come to that later.) A sweet spot can happen in a romantic relationship, a business partnership, a politician's reign, the life of a club or a group's friendship. It signals that time when all the ducks are in a row, when the stars are in alignment, and when the gods are smiling.

As noted, a sweet spot is typically associated with sport: It can last an instant, such as the perfect meeting of boot and ball when a striker takes a pressure penalty. It's the endorphin hit that a runner experiences midway through a long run, but which disappears if she runs too far or too fast. But it can be unrelated to sport and last for decades, or even centuries, as in the life of a culture like the Mayans of Central America, or the Moghuls of India. The sweet spot, despite its implied brevity, can be more than just a brief point in time.

A sweet spot can include the environment, a situation or a population. It's even encapsulated at the world level in James Lovelock's sweeping concept of Gaia, which invokes the notion of the earth as a living responsive system eternally struggling to maintain its ecospherical sweet spot against the pressures pulling it to over- and under-equilibrium.

To summarise, life's sweet spots form a diverse pattern. They can be big or small, brief or enduring, frequent or infrequent, suddenly or gradually occurring—and suddenly or gradually ceasing—and consecutive or simultaneous. The key point is that, although often difficult to objectify or define, they *do* exist, and are potent influences on human endeavour.

Humans appear to have less capacity than other organisms, however, to sense the end of a sweet spot, and hence tend to overshoot the time at which appropriate change may be made to gain the full benefits of the sweet spot experience. It's human nature to want to milk every last bit of pleasure from a situation. So we seek to *maximise* rather than *optimise* any experience, and in doing so, accelerate its demise. This is exemplified by the well-known Peter Principle, where an individual is inclined to rise in a work environment to his or her level of incompetence in search of an elusive sweeter spot, thus increasing the chances of meeting his or her personal Waterloo—that is, the dramatic end of the sweet spot where their job and abilities were in synch.

There is evidence to suggest that this point—the sweet spot—has now been reached, and possibly surpassed, in relation to the aspects of human prosperity that are the subject of this book: health, economic growth and greenhouse gas saturation leading to climate change. It is our belief that these apparently diverse sweet spots are related, and that it is important to recognise how this relationship occurs so that we can prevent the problems of overshoot.

Of course, economic growth, prosperity and human health have been intimately and positively related throughout history and, in particular, over the past 200 or so years since the beginnings of the Industrial Revolution. But in our opinion the relentless emphasis on economic growth has led to the sweet spots for both environmental wellbeing and human health being overshot. Obesity is a sign of this—when the sweet spot for human health ends as a consequence of *too much* economic growth, obesity begins. Climate change is also related to this. When waste emissions into the atmosphere from over-consumption driven by excess economic growth surpass the ability of environmental 'sinks' to soak them up, environmental disruption—an overshooting of the environmental sweet spot—is the outcome.

Our measure of economic wellbeing—gross domestic product (GDP), or the value of goods and services produced and traded in a given time—clearly has the potential to clash with any measure of human wellbeing, because, for example, around 9 per cent of GDP is made up of cigarette, alcohol and drug sales. So the more of these we consume, the healthier the economy becomes, even as our physical health may suffer proportionately. Yet despite many distinguished writers warning of the dangers of unfettered economic growth, and the hippie generation of the 1960s and 1970s protesting against over-population, pollution, resource scarcity and consequent world catastrophe, the potential clash has been ignored or downplayed by economists and governments since the 1980s. The discovery of new oil, an invigorated debate against birth control by the major religions and a dumbing down of discussion by politicians and corporations stung by the successful public reaction against the Vietnam War have put a lid on any thought that we may have surpassed our collective sweet spot.

More recently, the overshooting of the sweet spot has been linked to new findings relating to the human immune system which is now thought to play a much more direct part in the development of modern chronic diseases such as heart disease, Type 2 diabetes, respiratory diseases and many different forms of cancer, for which obesity is often seen as a cause. All these chronic diseases have a lifestyle or environmental base, influenced primarily by relentless economic growth. Now, despite our earlier belief that immunity plays an insignificant role in the development of *chronic* disease (although it obviously plays a vital role in *acute* infectious diseases, or injury), it seems that the human immune system has evolved to react to aspects of behaviour and the environment, generated by rapid economic growth, to which it is unaccustomed.

In failing to appreciate the link between disturbances of the immune system and *chronic* disease, we may have been sidetracked by the worldwide interest in obesity, which has been described as 'collateral damage in the battle for modernity', the 'unintended, but unavoidable consequence' of economic progress,' and 'simply a natural and inevitable biological response to living in a consumer-oriented democracy'. Obesity may not be a disease, as we have been led to believe, but a signal. It is a signal not only that something *might* be wrong healthwise in an individual (and therefore other risk factors need checking), but also that, when in epidemic proportions, something *definitely* is wrong in the broader environment in which the individual lives.

Obesity is the canary in the coalmine that should alert us to structural problems in society. At a metaphorical level, it is also a signal that we have reached the end of a sweet spot in human history, that, like Cinderella, we have stayed too long at the ball (as also indicated by accompanying and related environmental problems such as climate change), and that if we don't take this as a warning, all our carriages may be turned into pumpkins.

This is not to suggest that obesity is not important. However it may not be obesity *per se* but the things which can cause obesity—factors in our Western environment and lifestyle—which should be our prime cause of concern in looking at the big picture. These factors include access to energy-dense processed foods, energy-saving technology, high rates of stress and depression, and inadequate sleep—all of which are driven by economic growth. By applying an epidemiological (or population-wide) approach to these factors we are able to deduce the real cause of the problem—in essence, the cause of the causes—which in our view is unrestrained economic growth, for its own sake.

This doesn't imply a conspiracy, but there is little doubt that in the current economic environment it is in the best interests of governments (of all persuasions), as well as big business, both of which are beholden to the growth paradigm, for individuals to see obesity as merely the product of sloth and gluttony, and hence as solely an individual responsibility. This allows—in fact encourages—a continuation of the status quo where consumption is maintained (whether over-consumption of fattening foods and entertainment and effort-saving technology or consumption of products and services for weight loss) in order to prop up a dying economic paradigm—the imperative of growth.

Yet while obesity may be joked about because it superficially affects only the individual, it is harder to be humorous about the more global effects of over-consumption, such as climate change and species and resource extinction, which are paradoxically linked with increases in obesity through the same drive for unlimited growth. It is the coming together of these factors that demands a greater attention to the true causes of obesity and other modern chronic diseases if we are to deal with the problems of overshooting our sweet spots effectively.

CHAPTER 2
OBESITY: ITS PART IN OUR DOWNFALL

'Any important disease whose causality is murky, and for which treatment is ineffectual, tends to be awash in significance.'

SUSAN SONTAG, *ILLNESS AS METAPHOR*

Looking back at the 1950s and 1960s, when both of us were growing up, one thing is clear: there were few fat people and, in particular, very few fat children. The occasional overweight child typically came from a family where one or other parent or a sibling was of similar appearance.

It was also clear to us that humans, like all mammals, *could* get fat, given the right conditions. Obesity among the rich and powerful, for example, had long been a sign to the masses of just that—being rich and powerful—and still is in some parts of the globe. One African king who developed a taste for such symbolism is reputed to have fed his many queens cream and milk until they became so fat they had to be rolled to their conjugal duties. Still, for the vast amount of human history, the struggle for survival has meant that the majority of humans have essentially remained relatively lean, just as during our childhoods midway through the twentieth century.

Fast forward to today: not only are at least 20 per cent of Australian children under the age of twelve and 30 per cent under the age of eighteen in developed countries such as Australia now classified as overweight or obese, but at least one in three, and possibly as many as one in two, born in this millennium will go on to develop Type 2 diabetes, the classic 'fat' disease, in his or her lifetime. Among adults, the percentage regarded as overweight or obese is as high as 68 per cent in men and 56 per cent in women. This is from a base of less than 10 per cent for both sexes in the mid 1950s. Type 2 diabetes rates, which typically lag behind obesity, are now at 7 per cent of the population with a further 15 per cent qualifying as pre-diabetic, and likely to become diabetic in the next ten years.

We can immediately dismiss the notion that this is because we are living longer and diabetes is a disease of the aged. Type 2 diabetes, which is undoubtedly caused by the environment and behaviour (although not always by obesity, as we will see), is increasingly common in adolescents. Type 2 diabetes rates have increased proportionately in all ages, from youth to the elderly. And all of this has happened in the course of the last forty years. To see why this may be so, we have only to look at developing countries.

It's been known for some time that as a country develops economically its populace becomes fatter. This is not unexpected, as we are just a type of animal. And like cattle in a good paddock, it's easy to store energy in the form of fat in the good times, in preparation for future bad times that evolution has determined are likely to occur. However, unlike other animals, our mental capacity allows us to make a choice. So while the rich, upper classes become fattest in the early stages of development, and the working classes, who are still doing just that—physically working, with scant financial resources for over-eating relative to their energy expenditure—stay lean, the reverse occurs as development progresses. With education about the dangers of fatness, social pressure (at least in Western societies) and the means to stay lean, those of upper socio-economic status—well, the women at least—are able to reduce their body fatness. Meanwhile, without such education, and with growing access to the fruits of development, such as energy-dense processed foods, low relative food prices and effort-saving machinery like the motor car, lower socio-economic status groups increase the country's average body weight.

The shift in average weights is also affected by differences in physiology between genders and ages. As women are more important to the survival of the species because of their ability to bear children, Mother Nature has provided mechanisms through which women gain and store fat more readily than men, in order to survive those potential lean times. Similarly, as physical capacity decreases with ageing, it is advantageous for older animals—and humans—to be able to store energy more readily to compete against the young bucks who are quicker to the source of food. So it's not unexpected that the first group of humans to get fat in the early stages of the good paddock provided by economic advancement are women of child-bearing age; second are adult men; third are adolescents and fourth are juveniles. In a short period from a base of almost no obesity in the 1950s to today, developed countries such as the US, Australia, the UK, much of Europe and even some developing countries have reached stage 4 of the fattening process: children, as well as adults and adolescents, have become obese.

At the other extreme of economic development are the underdeveloped countries of much of Africa and many countries in South-East Asia, where the population lives to an average age of around forty-five, and is burdened by infectious diseases. Until recently, there was little incidence of chronic diseases (which have been called the 'diseases of modernity'), such as heart disease, Type 2 diabetes and cancers, and almost no obesity, except among the very wealthy, as in the early stages of development in Western countries. Unfortunately, these developing countries are now being hit by a double whammy. With easier access to Western fast foods and technology, parts of the population are becoming obese, sometimes in the midst of malnutrition. Children eating energy-dense but nutrient-poor processed foods, who are also less active as a result of technology, are becoming *over*-nourished, but, because of the poor quality of their food, they are also *mal*nourished, and burdened with the disease consequences of both extremes.

Somewhere in the middle are the rapidly developing countries, the best examples of which are India and China. Although China is now officially regarded as an economy 'in transition', using modern economic parlance, it has only really been so since the mid 1990s. Anyone visiting both the then underdeveloped China and the significantly Westernised Hong Kong before that time would have been struck by the huge differences in obesity levels between the essentially genetically homogenous populations. Figures quoted by the international obesity expert Professor Phillip James in 1980, show that overweight and obesity in the mainland Chinese population was then at a level less than 5 per cent. Since that time, however, until the global financial crisis of 2007–08, growth rates of the economy exceeded 10 per cent per annum and the levels of overweight and obesity jumped rapidly to around 22 per cent of the population. And while a lag time for the accompanying Type 2 diabetes outbreak might be expected, by 2007–08, an estimated 9.5 per cent of the population was already diagnosed as having the disease, and an extra 14.4 per cent was pre-diabetic. Based on current rates of development, it is predicted that an extra 40 million of China's current population of 1.37 billion will become diabetic in the next ten years. In other parts of Asia, the diabetes epidemic is also skyrocketing in line with rapid economic growth. It rose from 3 per cent in the 1970s to 12 per cent in 2000 among Indian adults, and from 2.3 per cent to 6.8 per cent in rural Bangladesh. Around 60 per cent of the expected growth in Type 2 diabetes cases worldwide, from 240 million to 380 million in 2025, is expected to come from Asia, the part of the world with the fastest current rate of economic growth.

Obesity results from an energy imbalance, where energy refers to calories, or kilojoules. An imbalance, and hence a build-up of fat, can occur as a result of an excess intake of food or drink, a decrease in energy expended through physical activity, or a combination of increased intake and decreased activity. In the past it was thought that this was explained by a simple equation: weight = energy in − energy out. However, in the 1990s it became clear that this equation is likely to work only in an environment not influenced by 'feedback'. Thus, as American obesity researcher J.P. Flatt reasoned, under such an equation a 70kg man at age 80 who had eaten just one extra slice of toast and butter for breakfast throughout his life would instead weigh 170kg. Clearly this is extremely unlikely and shows the absurdity of the average 'diet of the week', where calorie counting is supposed to lead to a fixed amount of weight loss among different individuals.

As any health-conscious couple on the same weight loss regime will know, *he* will typically strip off the kilos with little effort, while *she* will struggle for every gram. You'll see the same differences in ability to lose weight between (and sometimes within) families, between different ethnic groups, at different ages, and after different life stages and events (giving up smoking being a key one). The static paradigm obviously doesn't work and it's about time we acknowledged this.

In 1997, we devised a more dynamic formula for body weight, taking into account a range of influences that affect any biological organism.

In the first place we suggested that body weight, in a biological being, is never static, but can change weekly, daily or hourly, like sand on a beach, which comes and goes depending on the state of the waves and weather. Energy intake and expenditure *are* common pathways, but they are influenced by biology (genetics, age, gender), behaviour (e.g., whether one is a restrained eater or not) and the environment (the modern industrial environment versus the classical hunter–gatherer situation). Most importantly, all of these factors can be moderated by physiological adjustments. A decrease in energy intake (food consumption), for example, especially a large decrease, can create a physical response to dampen the impact of that energy decrease (loss of food) on weight loss and thus improve the chances of long-term survival in case of famine. So for example, a 100kg person who loses 10% of his body weight, might have a 12% drop in his metabolic rate, or the rate at which the body burns energy, thus making it harder to continue losing weight.

Genetics also has a significant role. But this role must be seen in the context of a complicated interaction with the environment. As Dr George Bray, a leading expert in the field of obesity has noted: 'With obesity, genetics loads the gun, but environment pulls the trigger.' Genes are therefore likely to have the biggest influence on the development of obesity among the very small number of individuals with a large genetic predisposition for storing fat. This explains the rarity of obesity amongst hunter–gatherers, tribesmen and those struggling to eke out an existence in poor countries. But in a different type of environment, where energy-dense foods and effort-saving machinery are readily available, such as in the modern post-industrial world, minimal genetic predisposition (and virtually all humans have this) can lead to over-fatness.

For a long time it was thought that obesity was a limited genetic phenomenon, that just a few genes dictated whether someone becomes fat or not in a given environment. The advent of sophisticated genetic research techniques showed that there are perhaps hundreds of genes that can have an influence on body weight. Suffice it to say that while genes do obviously play a part in the susceptibility of particular individuals to become obese, they have been over-emphasised as the primary cause of the problem. A figure of 40–60 per cent of obesity being explained by genetics is an often misquoted statistic. In fact, if all of the findings of the research on genes which determine obesity are combined, they only explain a few per cent of the variations in body mass index.

While the new model we devised for body weight (see Figure 2.1) explains individual variations in body weight and caters for genetic differences and abnormalities, perhaps its biggest benefit is in the understanding it provides of increases in population levels of obesity. We've previously suggested that obesity is a 'natural response to an unnatural ('obesogenic') environment', rather than, as had previously been thought, 'an unnatural response to a natural environment'. While to the unitiated it seems that obesity is a product of individual sloth and gluttony stemming from a lack of personal discipline, the experiences in different economies (developed, developing and underdeveloped) indicate that it is the environment, and (as we will see) economic growth in particular, that lies behind the worldwide obesity epidemic. It is our belief, after decades of trying to understand the causes of the problem, that increased population levels of obesity are a marker of economic growth having overshot its sweet spot. This also correlates with increases in environmental degradation and the rise of problems such as climate change, which could ultimately lead to the next world sour spot (see Chapter 7). As we will see, there is also a sweet spot for levels of fatness in the body: too little is dangerous, as is too much. Obesity, at the population level, signals having collectively overshot this particular sweet spot for body fat. Should we be concerned about this as a cause of disease? We'll get back to that after a short diversion into the nature and physiology of fat.

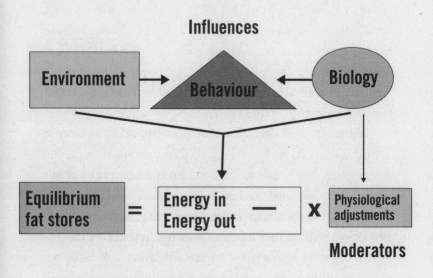

FIGURE 2.1 AN ECOLOGICAL MODEL OF OBESITY

While energy balance is the key, this is constantly affected by a range of influences and moderators, making the equation of
weight = energy in – energy out overly simplistic.

CHAPTER 3
GOOD FAT VERSUS BAD FAT

'When the facts change, I change my mind. What do you do, sir?'

JOHN MAYNARD KEYNES

Throughout history, obesity has never been common among the masses. It has existed in select individuals, as testified by ancient artefacts such as the Venus of Willendorf, an 11 cm statuette of a woman with a large waist and pendulous breasts, found in central Europe and dating back 23,000 years. Some Roman and Greek potentates were also massively obese, as were small numbers of (usually privileged) individuals over the ensuing millennia. Although sometimes deaths occurred directly as a result of obesity, such as that of the King of Cyrene who 'weighted down with monstrous masses of flesh . . . choked himself to death' in 258 BCE, there has long been a view that there is also a more subtle link between obesity and ill-health. Hippocrates, for example, noted that 'sudden death is more common in those who are naturally fat than in the lean', and the Roman physician Galen went so far as to describe two types of obesity: 'moderate' and 'immoderate'; the former considered as 'natural', and not a cause of disease, and the latter, 'morbid', with a clear link to disease, hinting at a disparity that is still accepted in some form today.

The first formal acceptance of obesity as a health problem came in the late nineteenth century when US actuaries working on a new formula for body mass based on height and weight, as calculated by the Belgian mathematician Adolphe Quetelet, found an association with death rates. (Quetelet's index is now known as Body Mass Index or BMI. BMI = weight in kilos divided by height in metres^2.) This provided some statistical support for Hippocrates' musings. Still, the levels of obesity in the population were not sufficient to cause alarm in an era characterised by a relatively short life span, most usually influenced by a preponderance of infectious diseases. Also, because the focus was on body mass and disease, it provided only a rough estimate of risk at the individual level, as it still does today. For example, it discriminates against certain body types, such as the short, muscular mesomorphic build—usually males—and the elderly, who tend to 'shrink' with age and thus increase in BMI with no gain in weight. Some time ago, players from a first-grade rugby league side playing at the top level in the Sydney competition approached one of us about a problem with their team doctor. Playing an 80-minute, intense, highly physical game, rugby league players are among the fittest athletes on the planet, typically with 3–5 per cent body fat, but often mesomorphic in build, as muscular bulk is an asset in body contact sport. All had been told by the team GP, based on their BMI scores, that they needed to lose weight.

It was not until the 1940s that the French endocrinologist Dr Jean Vague, drawing on Galen's observation of 'natural' and 'unnatural' obesities, deduced that some sites of body fat storage seem to be more predictive of disease (particularly heart disease) than others. According to Vague, 'android' or apple-shaped individuals with abdominal obesity, such as is more common in men and post-menopausal women, seemed to more often meet an early demise than 'gynoid', or pear-shaped individuals with greater fat stores around the hips and buttocks (usually pre-menopausal women). Subsequent experts have suggested that these latter fat stores, which are physiologically more difficult to reduce than the former, have a function in survival of the species, as they provide energy stores for women to last the nine months of pregnancy and beyond, in case of a famine.

Because it was originally published in French, Vague's 1947 revelation went largely unheeded in the English-speaking world, and particularly the US, until the obesity epidemic began to germinate in the 1970s and 1980s. Subsequent research, particularly in Scandinavia, confirmed Vague's theories by showing reduced mortality and morbidity rates in gynoid-shaped females, irrespective of BMI. This gave rise to the measure of waist-to-hip ratio (WHR), and then just waist circumference (WC) alone as a predictive measure of disease risk. Caucasian males who had a WHR of >1.00 and a WC of more than 102 cm were deemed to be at increased risk of metabolic disease compared with those under these levels. The comparative measures for Caucasian females were 0.90

and 94 cm. Although WHR measures are probably consistent between ethnic groups, and WHR cut-offs consistent across ethnic groups, confusion still reigns about comparative cut-offs for WC for groups other than Caucasians. With Asians and Indians the respective figures have been proposed to be 8–10 cm less than for Caucasians, and for Pacific Islanders somewhat more. Norms are still being tested for other ethnic groups. Still, as a result of the confirmed role of abdominal fat in disease, the tool for measuring waist size—a tape measure!—is increasingly important in medical practice.

The rapid increase in the number of obese individuals in the Western world throughout the 1980s and 1990s led to further investigation of body fat stores and scientists discovered forms of fat that had previously not been recognised. New technology enabled the imaging of internal fat around organs such as the kidneys, liver and stomach. This became known as visceral adipose tissue (VAT), and in the early 1990s was found to be more dangerous than subcutaneous adipose tissue (SAT)—the type of fat we 'see' on obese people. Although related to SAT, and therefore more likely in someone with a large waist, VAT was found to be quite high in some lean individuals and to be relatively low in some fat ones. It was also found to be associated with metabolic abnormalities, particularly insulin resistance and Type 2 diabetes. VAT was soon thought to be possibly the main link between obesity and disease.

In pre-industrial days, the diseases linked with obesity were limited to heart disease and conditions such as gout and sleep apnoea, which were seen as accompaniments to corpulence as far back as the Roman Empire. The number of recognised obesity-related diseases, though, began to rise with more sophisticated medical research and a greater understanding of different diseases. Type 2 diabetes, for example, which was almost unknown in pre-industrial societies, began to take off in the US, Australia and Europe in the 1970s with the rise of obesity (a time which also marks the acceleration of global warming and world economic growth, the coincidence of which will soon be shown).

Among a growing list of other metabolic disorders associated with obesity are stroke, just about all cancers (breast, endometrial and colon, in particular), gall bladder disease, polycystic ovaries, impaired fertility and skin complications. More mechanical problems linked to obesity include breathlessness, asthma, daytime sleepiness, reflux, stress incontinence, cellulitis, arthritis and other musculoskeletal problems. And while general obesity is predictive of many of these, VAT is an even more powerful predictor of metabolic complications.

Around the turn of the millennium, scientists started to understand more clearly the nature of VAT, or metabolically dangerous fat. To appreciate this, we need to take a brief tour into the basic physiology of fat.

Fat exists in specialised cells in the body known as adipocytes. An adipocyte has all the inner workings of other cells in the body, but also includes a lipid or fat pool, a form of reserve energy in the cell.

The average human body has around 30–50 billion of these cells, which expand and contract with the intake or release of fat according to the energy balance of the individual.

Most gains in body weight come from the expansion of these individual cells, which occur in most parts of the body. Once a fat cell is full up, new cells may spring up from baby fat cells (pre-adipocytes) which are a form of stem cell lying between existing fat cells waiting to be called into life. Sometimes, though, when the existing cells are full, extra fat 'spills over' from the full fat cells into other parts of the body instead, forming what is known as ectopic fat stores—that is, storage of fat in non-adipose (fat) tissue.

One of the first areas to store this spillover fat is the liver, but excess fat also flows into the blood (raising blood lipids), into muscles (leading to intra-muscular fat), and into other organs, increasing visceral fat. For reasons not yet clear, but probably genetically based, some individuals start to spill over at a low level of overall body fat and some don't spill over even at a high level. In other words, a lean individual may experience significant spillover and an obese person experience very little. It seems counter-intuitive, but fat seems to be metabolically healthy—as long as it stays in the fat cells!

When it occurs, spillover acts a bit like boiling water in a saucepan. It can cause damage to anything it comes in contact with, and as we will see in the next chapter it can cause an increase in inflammation, both in the fat cell itself and throughout the rest of the body. Specifically how this spillover leads to chronic disease is not yet clear. Suffice it to say that some people seem to be able to increase their fat cell size or number, and therefore their total level of body fat—even to the point of being classified as obese—without any apparent health consequences. A lean, apparently healthy individual, on the other hand, may be limited in his or her fat cell expansion ability, and can suffer from numerous metabolic diseases and conditions at a low level of body fatness, and even with no apparent abdominal fat. In a recent Japanese study, individuals of roughly the same body weight, but with different amounts of VAT, or dangerous fat, were put on a weight loss program. Although about the same amount of weight was lost in both groups, more VAT was lost in the group that had the higher level of VAT in the first place, suggesting this is the first place that fat is lost when energy balance becomes negative.

So now the picture has become a little more complicated. Although there is increased disease risk associated with different locations of fat storage on the body, there can also be different health patterns within this, probably associated with genetic limitations to fat spillover. Figure 3.1 shows the various fat and health states and their approximate proportions for US adults.

All this suggests that obesity is usually, but not necessarily a risk factor for physical disease. In fact there appears to be a sweet spot for levels of body fatness within a range that is apparently optimal for good health. (In males a recommended percentage range of body fat for good health is 12–24 per cent of total body mass. In females the range is 15–35 per cent.) And while the bottom levels of this are probably relatively consistent for most people, the upper levels may vary according to the genetic predisposition for fat to spill over.

The fact that fat is healthy—up to a point—is supported by recent findings that up to one in three obese individuals and one in two of the overweight have no current metabolic problems associated with their weight, while possibly as many as one in four lean individuals do (see Figure 3.1). Of course

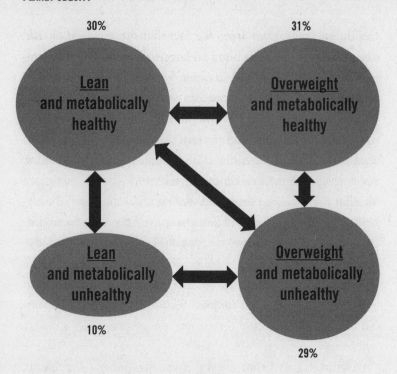

FIGURE 3.1 LINKS BETWEEN FAT AND HEALTH

Metabolic health or ill-health can exist in either the lean or obese in proportions of the total US population represented roughly by the size of the ovals.

this is no proof of causality, and even indicates a relationship between obesity and ill-health, as the relative risk increases with increased body weight. However, this is not as high as might be expected. Also, it should be noted that a high proportion of smokers don't get lung cancer, and a proportion of people who don't smoke do (although this is very small). But this doesn't take away from the fact that the *population risk* of getting lung cancer is highly related to smoking in the community. Similarly, obesity, in some form, is correlated with a range of different chronic diseases and appears to be causally related. So we should not discount obesity prevention and weight loss as being unimportant for good health. Yet the analysis to date suggests obesity is not *always*, and sometimes not even *usually*, the direct cause of chronic disease, suggesting that the focus for intervention might be taken off obesity *per se*. But if obesity shouldn't always be the main focus for chronic disease reduction, what should?

CHAPTER 4

THE ROLE OF INFLAMMATION

'If we want to know why diabetes and other diseases are on the rise . . . we need to focus less on the mere fact that our weight is increasing and more on the question of why our weight is increasing. In other words, we need to listen to what our growing weight is telling us.'

J. ERIC OLIVER, *FAT POLITICS*

In 1993, Gokhan Hotamisligil, a young Turkish doctor in Harvard University's Department of Genetics and Complex Diseases, noted a hitherto unrecognised phenomenon: that some obesity seems to be accompanied by a form of low-grade inflammation, similar but different in scale to that which develops as an immune response to acute infections and wounds. On the basis of this, Hotamisligil suggested that obesity may cause disease as a result of a chronic inflammatory reaction. If this was true, it might help to explain the physiological link between obesity and chronic disease, like heart disease, Type 2 diabetes, respiratory disease and many forms of cancer. To understand the implications of this, we need to again take a step back to examine the process of inflammation and its role in protection against disease.

Inflammation is a reaction by the immune system to restrict the spread of a potential disease, when the body suffers injury or invasion by a microbial organism such as a bacteria or virus. As explained by immunologist Dr John Dwyer in his book *The Body at War*, the mammalian immune system is like an army, with specialist 'warriors' designed to recognise, surround, delay, destroy and then mop up the detritus of anything foreign entering the body with the potential to disturb its normally healthy equilibrium. Inflammation occurs in the early stages of invasion, and in classical infection is usually a large and acute response designed to keep the attackers hemmed in until help arrives. A defensive 'wall' is built up by pro-inflammatory 'warriors' which can rise by 100 or 200 times the normal level following an infection such as pneumonia. Other 'warrior' molecules are anti-inflammatory and help break down the defensive wall once a threat has passed.

Hotamisligil and his team discovered that there is a different type of inflammation associated with obesity. This varies from the classical inflammatory response in a number of ways: first, it causes only a small rise in the pro-inflammatory 'warriors' discussed above (3- to 6-fold versus 100-fold); secondly, it results in chronic, rather than acute change; thirdly, it has its effects in the lining of the blood vessels throughout the body rather than in local organs; fourthly, its foreign agents, or 'invaders', are relatively subtle and are known as 'inducers';

and finally, because it is chronic or long term, it appears to perpetuate rather than resolve a disease by changing normal metabolic functioning. Because this type of inflammation is associated with the metabolic system, Hotamisligil called it 'metaflammation', to distinguish it from classical inflammation. To sum up, classical inflammation results in a large and acute inflammatory response, which is usually resolved, returning the body to normal. Metaflammation, on the other hand, results in much less of an inflammatory reaction, but can result in chronic changes to the metabolism and chronic disease.

As a result of Hotamisligil's work, it is now thought that metaflammation is a link between obesity and chronic disease. But metaflammation is also caused by factors other than obesity and is sometimes found in the absence of obesity. Scientists are only just beginning to identify the 'inducers' of metaflammation (and hence much chronic disease) other than obesity, and have discovered that some of them cause metaflammation when they exist in small amounts or in excess, but have the opposite (anti-inflammatory) effects when they exist in moderation. Being inactive, for example, which one might expect to be unhealthy, does cause an increase in pro-inflammatory markers throughout the blood. Exercise, on the other hand, which might be expected to be a positive health habit, seems to also cause a pro-inflammatory reaction (bad) in the early stages of an exercise program, but an anti-inflammatory effect (good) as fitness develops. However, if exercise is extended at a high level of intensity over time, such as in a series of marathon type events, the effect is pro-inflammatory—that is, too much exercise leads to metaflammation.

Different amounts of alcohol in the diet have a similar effect: a moderate amount is good, but too little or too much is not so good for metaflammation. More specifically, a moderate daily intake of any form of alcohol (up to 250 ml a day) can be anti-inflammatory, whereas bingeing, or drinking an excessive amount in any 24-hour period, can be pro-inflammatory. As protection against metaflammation appears to be provided by anti-oxidants in alcohol, drinks like red wine, which have a high proportion of anti-oxidants, have the most beneficial effect, but all alcohol seems to have some benefit if taken in moderation.

Similarly, as might be expected, good, healthy food is anti-inflammatory, or at least has a neutral effect on the development of metaflammation when eaten in moderation. But too much healthy food can be bad for you—as far as inflammation goes. The response to a nutrient overload from a very big meal at one sitting, for example, even if made up of all healthy foods, can be pro-inflammatory. On the other hand, even a small amount of unhealthy food (particularly if it is high in saturated fat) can be metaflammatory, at least over the short term. If this is eaten regularly in large meals over the long term, the effects can be chronically metaflammatory and unhealthy. If the techniques for measuring such an effect were available when Morgan Spurlock made his movie Super Size Me, about eating high-energy fast foods exclusively for an entire month, it's almost certain that his unhealthy status would have included a chronic level of metaflammation.

But it is not just too little or too much of a particular inducer that can cause metaflammation and increase one's risk of chronic disease. There are other factors that can bring about this effect even in moderate amounts. Balancing this, there are factors that can cause an anti-inflammatory reaction, or at least a reduction of inflammation to a neutral response. A few years ago, one of us (GE) set out with some colleagues and students to identify these, to try to detect a pattern beyond mere obesity. The team listed all those inducers identified so far as being either pro- or anti-inflammatory for metaflammation as shown in Table 4.1.

It's disconcertingly clear that none of the pro-inflammatory stimuli set out in the table are microbial 'invaders', as is the case in the classical inflammatory response. Instead, all are related in some way to lifestyle or the environment.

Obesity, as an outcome of many of these behaviours, is just one of a number of inducers of metaflammation. Even in the case of factors causing obesity, such as too much food, there is an indication that obesity doesn't have to be an outcome for metaflammation to occur. Several studies have shown changes in inflammatory markers owing to dietary intake in the absence of weight gain. As with alcohol and exercise, discussed above, fasting for more than about 48 hours (the opposite of nutrient overload) can have a metaflammatory effect, and this can be in the presence of weight *loss*! Other nutrient factors which cause metaflammation are fast foods and a Western style diet, saturated and trans fats in foods, fructose- (fruit sugar) and glucose- (cane sugar) rich foods and drinks, excess alcohol and refined or processed carbohydrate in the diet.

Non-nutrient inducers, apart from, and often independent of weight gain, include inactivity as well as excess activity, inadequate sleep, smoking, stress, anxiety, depression, vitamin D deficiency and a generally unhealthy modern lifestyle.

TABLE 4.1 THE EFFECTS OF LIFESTYLE ON CHRONIC DISEASE

PRO-INFLAMMATORY STIMULI	ANTI-INFLAMMATORY STIMULI*
Obesity	**Weight loss**
Nutrition	**Nutrition**
– excessive energy intake	– fruits, vegetables
– saturated fatty acids	– nuts
– 'trans' fats	– high mono-unsaturated fatty acid
– high glycaemic load diet	– fish, fish oils
– high GI foods	– tea, green tea
– fructose	– garlic
– refined carbohydrate	– herbs and spices
– low N3/N6 ratio	– capsaicin
– excess salt	– lean game meats
– excessive alcohol	– vinegar
– high fat Western style diet	– low GI foods
– fast food	– high fibre diet
Inactivity	– olive oil
Excessive exercise	– grapes, raisins
Smoking	– dark chocolate
Sleep deprivation	– high N3:N6 ratio
Stress/Anxiety/Depression	– red wine, moderate alcohol intake
Low humidity	– Mediterranean diet
Air pollution	– calorie restriction
Sick building syndrome	**Physical activity**
	Smoking cessation
	Intensive lifestyle change

* or 'neutral' when compared to its opposite pro-inflammatory form

In the environment, air pollution, low humidity, and even 'sick building syndrome' also seem to be metaflammatory. An Italian doctor and pharmacologist, Dr Donatella Zappulla, has recently suggested that increased carbon dioxide in the bloodstream, which can be caused by exposure to greater levels of carbon dioxide in the air, may also be inflammatory—an interesting finding considering the rise of carbon in the atmosphere which, as we will see, is also implicated in climate change.

Already, you might be starting to detect a pattern in relation to the stimuli causing metaflammation. As a clue, it's worth pointing out that the immune system reacts to inducers with which it has not evolved and does not have either an innate immunity or has not developed an acquired immunity.

Even a casual observation of the anti-inflammatory responses (or neutral responses) shown on the right-hand side of the table reveals that all of them have been around for a long time throughout human history. Most of the pro-inflammatory inducers identified on the left-hand side of Table 4.1, on the other hand, are familiar only to modern humans, and have probably been around only since the time of the industrial revolution of the late nineteenth century. Hence, there has been little time for the human immune system to adapt to them, resulting in a low-grade, defensive inflammatory reaction (metaflammation). The human immune system is reacting to our twenty-first century lifestyle and environment in a fashion similar to the way in which the immune system has developed over hundreds of thousands of years to respond to a microbial invader like a bacteria, virus, fungus or other pathogen.

With the vision of hindsight, this makes sense. The genus *homo erectus*, or the most recent human-like life form, has existed for possibly 2 million years. *Homo sapiens*, the modern form of human being, have been around for over 100,000 years, and in that time have adapted to a wide range of natural foods (fruits, vegetables, nuts, seeds etc.), environments and behaviours. Over that time, a certain level of physical activity was required for humans to hunt or collect enough food to survive, and also to escape from predators. Such activity has become associated in the selection process with a healthy metabolism. The post-industrial revolution environment, which has given rise to processed, high-fat, energy-dense foods and energy-saving technologies, has only existed for around 200 years and still requires extra effort from humans to achieve a level of physical activity recognised by the body as normal. Little wonder components of this environment seem foreign to the body in a way that sets up a defensive immune reaction.

A possible point of contention with this theory concerns the physiological agent to which the immune system reacts. How and why does the body react to different elements of the modern Western lifestyle. In the case of food, which is ingested, this is not hard to explain. Saturated fat, which is the nutrient perhaps most widely agreed by scientists to be metaflammatory, was much less common throughout evolutionary history. Saturated fats come mainly from animal meats and are highest in animals that are confined, rather than allowed to range freely in their natural environment. The farming of animals for food by confining them and feeding them foods to which they are naturally unaccustomed (e.g., corn) is a relatively recent historical event. It is not hard, therefore, to see how derivatives of saturated fat can act as an inducer to the immune system to cause the low-level build-up of an inflammatory defence reaction. Smoking and air pollution as inflammatory inducers can also be understood because of the ingestion by the body of foreign particulate matter and noxious gases. It would seem more difficult, though, to explain the inducer effects of inactivity or inadequate sleep. However, research suggests that this may result from the chronic production of stress-related hormones such as cortisol, which, when hanging around in the body long enough, interfere with the immune defence reaction and result in a pro-inflammatory response.

On the other side of the ledger (and table), some foods and behaviours that are anti-inflammatory may have only been used by certain races, not the total world population, for an extended period of time. How could humans in general, then, develop an anti-inflammatory reaction from that inducer? The Chinese, for example have consumed tea for at least 3500 years, but it was only introduced widely to Europe by the British in the seventeenth century. With such a short time span for genetic modification, how could tea have an anti-inflammatory effect in Caucasians? The answer could lie in the *ingredients* of the product rather than the product *per se*. Tea is rich in a type of anti-oxidant called polyphenol, also common in other plants, such as many fruits, vegetables, and spices, long known to Caucasians.

Similarly, the Mediterranean diet, which involves a high intake of seafood, pasta, fruits, vegetables, nuts and olive oil, has been well publicised as a healthy form of eating for all humans, not just those from southern Europe where the diet has been eaten for centuries. Although this hasn't yet been tested, we would argue that the Nordic diet, the Australian

Aboriginal diet, the Hunza diet, the Okinawa diet, or indeed any diet eaten traditionally by inhabitants of a particular region since before the advent of food processing, battery feeding of animals and genetic engineering of plants, would be as equally healthy and anti-inflammatory as the Mediterranean diet, and equally appropriate for all humans, due to their shared emphasis on fresh, natural, organic-style produce.

All this suggests that weight gain and obesity may be neither necessary nor sufficient alone to explain the increase in chronic disease in recent times. Indeed while some metaflammatory inducers may be linked to obesity, many inducers can lead to inflammation independent of obesity (e.g., smoking, over-exercise). Figure 4.1 shows how this can work, and suggests that it is aspects of the modern lifestyle, as much as the obesity that may or may not result from this, which are the driving forces behind the chronic disease epidemic.

Many people reading this may feel relieved by these statements. Overweight or obesity is not due to wilful overeating and indolence, it seems, but is due more to passive overconsumption of food and low activity levels in response to our modern Western environment. Eating too much and moving too little may still be the issue, but this has become the norm in a population encouraged to do so by the drive to consume, and feelings of guilt and misunderstanding about this experienced by many of those influenced by the modern environment may be misplaced and even counter-productive for good health. Obesity and overweight may also not necessarily lead to disease. However, this does not mean that obesity prevention and weight control should be ignored. Managing obesity is clearly still an issue, as processes to do this will also modify lifestyle factors causing metaflammation and other problems. (For example, increasing physical activity can improve sleep, decrease depression and so on.)

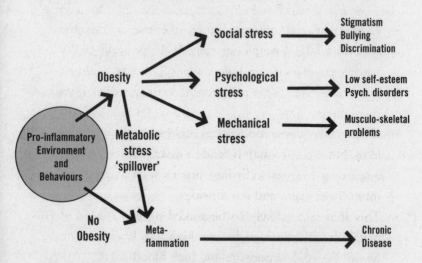

FIGURE 4.1 THE EFFECTS OF LIFESTYLE ON CHRONIC DISEASE

Lifestyle may or may not lead to obesity as shown by the arrows from the circle on the left, In turn, obesity may or may not lead to chronic disease (for reasons discussed in the text), or mechanical or psychological and social problems. However, some forms of obesity, or more importantly, the type of lifestyle behaviours that may or may not cause obesity, as shown along the bottom, can lead to chronic disease through metaflammation.

As pointed out in Chapter 3, and hopefully becoming clearer now, obesity is a sign that something *might* be metabolically awry in an individual. However, when obesity is in epidemic proportions, it is a sign that something *definitely* is wrong in the environment. Initiatives that identify the *population*, not the individual, as the unit of intervention are thus likely to have most impact on obesity and chronic disease.

Let's summarise where we have come from so far:

- Overweight and obesity are on the rise worldwide. Around 1 billion people, or roughly 15 per cent of the world's population, are now classified as overweight or obese. And there is no end in sight to the growth of the pandemic.
- Obesity may cause mechanical and psychosocial problems, but seems to mainly lead to disease when there is a spillover from fat cells into organs such as the liver, into other viscera and into muscles.
- This spillover is likely to be picked up in markers of metabolic ill-health including high fat levels in the blood, high blood pressure and high blood sugars.
- Rising population levels of obesity are a sign that something is awry in the modern Western lifestyle.
- This is supported by the fact that the prevalence of obesity varies significantly between countries at different stages of development.
- Obesity is also associated with a form of low-grade body-wide inflammation (metaflammation), which appears to be as much influenced by behavioural and environmental factors as by obesity itself, and which is the likely mediator of much chronic disease.

We'll now make the bold step of linking the rise in obesity with economic growth beyond a sweet spot in industrialised and rapidly industrialising countries. We'll then go on (in Chapter 6) to show how this also corresponds with an increase in environmental degradation and ultimately, climate change.

CHAPTER 5

HEALTH, 'ILLTH', ECONOMIC GROWTH AND THE SWEET SPOT

'. . . obesity is not so much the illness of an individual, no matter how greedy that person may be; it is the illness of the world that is feeding its hunger. And we will never overcome it until we are prepared to rethink, in depth, the ways in which we produce, sell and consume our food.'

FRANCIS DELPEUCH ET AL, GLOBESITY

In Chapter 2, the modern industrialised environment and the lifestyles emanating from this were suggested as factors behind the worldwide rise in obesity. We also hinted at economic growth being the prime reason our lifestyles have changed for the worse, and therefore the possible underlying cause of the obesity pandemic. This is a big call. To most economists and politicians the suggestion of a negative side to growth smacks of heresy, despite the fact that this was widely mooted by the early economists, such as John Stuart Mill and

J.M. Keynes, who were the originators of the modern growth system of economics.

It is not our intention to outline the technicalities of economic growth. For our purposes it is sufficient to understand that such a system, which was originally discussed as early as the eighteenth century by economist–philosophers such as Adam Smith and Thomas Malthus as well as Mill, is based on the notion of progressive increases in production and consumption in a society. In other words, it is necessary to produce, buy and sell more next year than this year, in order for a society to 'grow'. There is little consideration given by those who run the system to the fact that such growth is exponential and therefore ultimately limited, but it is driven to extremes in the meantime by any form of consumption that fuels the economic engine. As people's desires are met, new means of achieving growth are devised through the development of complicated credit systems, new advertising media, increasing specialisation, extended shopping hours and the promotion and consumption of unnecessary products. More and more consumption becomes necessary to keep the system on the rails, with little consideration of the effects on human or environmental welfare. As the system reaches capacity, governments are forced into a schizophrenic response favouring increasingly more irrelevant production while rationalising the effects on humanity of such production—obesity, pollution and so on.

One reason politicians take only half-hearted steps to reduce smoking, for example, is that tobacco farming, production and sales, as well as costs of treatment of tobacco-related illnesses, are all grist to the growth mill. In a perhaps more obvious way, obesity is dependent on over-consumption of food, drink and effort-saving technology; the fatter the population, the fatter the economy. This was cleverly illustrated by a spoof pitch on *The Gruen Transfer*, an ABC TV program on advertising in 2009. Asked to develop a campaign to reduce prejudice against obesity, one agency came up with an advertisement praising fat people as 'heroes' in the battle to reverse the 2008–9 global financial crisis because of their over-consumption of food. The catch phrase: 'Australia: Our success depends on your excess' sums up the modern conundrum.

Around the same time, the *Age* newspaper, on 13 May 2009, reporting on a health survey carried out in 2008 stated: 'As waistlines expand, so, too, does the cost to the taxpayer of caring for the increasing incidence of weight-related diabetes, heart disease and cancer. Obesity, therefore, is not just a burden on the individual, but on us all.'

A closer economic analysis of the impact of growing obesity rates, however, would show that while the taxpayer may be burdened, the economy is blessed, not just by the extra consumption causing the problem but by the health costs— read, economic benefits—in treating it.

A recent US study verifies this. Reporting in the journal *Health Affairs*, researchers calculated that the health costs for an obese individual are $1400 per year more than for a lean individual. This adds an extra $47 billion each year to the US economy, which is around 10 per cent of all health spending.

Looked at in this light, obesity is an economic godsend. Not only does it contribute to growth at the consumption end, but more and more it contributes throughout the weight-gain process. Food manufacturers, for example, can dramatically increase profitability, thereby adding to growth, by 'supersizing' servings while decreasing marginal costs. A standard serve at McDonald's in the 1950s included 72 g of fries and 200ml of Coca Cola. By 2001 it had increased to 205 g of fries and 950 ml of Coke. With increased sales of computer games, cars, the internet and other effort-saving devices, and more economic incentives not to move than to move, it's unlikely that the extra calories taken in here would be burned off through extra energy expenditure. Meanwhile, commercial weight loss companies reap the benefits of the increasingly corpulent 'lipo-warriors' spending more to save the economy. At the extreme end, surgeons and their allies reap the benefits of the $AU12,000–$15,000 fee for obesity surgery. (Surgery for obesity in the US, for example, increased ten-fold in the decade from 1995 to 2005, from 16,200 to 171,000 procedures.) The increase in one such surgical operation, laproscopic gastric banding, as measured by Medicare item numbers in Australia, from just a few in 1994 to around 14,000 in 2005 must be music to Treasury Department ears—possibly one reason it was promoted by a parliamentary inquiry such as the Australian Government's report *Weighing it Up*.

The nineteenth-century scholar John Ruskin, prominent in the early stages of the post-industrial revolution economic growth discussion, was the first to describe this paradox between economic and human wellbeing. He recognised that in the economic discussion of the time, no account had been taken of the production of objects that caused harm or were socially undesirable, but still had value in exchange. He referred to these as 'illth' objects, examples of which today might be cigarettes, illicit drugs and guns designed specifically to kill people.

Modern economists, who seek to drive the growth train further and faster, have typically ignored the concept of illth, even while cognisant that exponential growth of anything has obvious limitations. This is not to suggest, however, that growth *per se* is inherently bad. The proposition put here is that economic growth, like the growth of anything physical, has benefits to a point of maturity (its 'sweet spot'). But beyond that point there begin to develop diminishing or negative returns. As expressed by one writer: '. . . growth beyond maturity is either obesity or cancer.'

Before analysing this in detail, it's worth reconsidering the ultimate purpose of any economic system. This should be the advancement of human welfare, with all its connotations—environmental sustainability, biodiversity, equity and, of course, health which is our main consideration here. But human health and wellbeing are also intimately connected with ecological wellbeing. If James Lovelock's concept of 'Gaia', as the equilibrium of the whole biosphere is accepted (as it is becoming increasingly), our very existence can be seen to be dependent on the welfare of that living and interactive biosphere. And while growth, as measured in purely monetary terms, may run parallel to Gaia's welfare to a point, beyond that point there is likely to be a disconnect.

There is little doubt that in the past there has been a positive, almost perfect, correlation between growth and health. Growth has been validated by continuing improvements in death rates in all developing countries. The number of countries in which the average life expectancy is now more than 70 years, for example, has doubled over the last thirty years, in direct relationship with economic growth in those countries. There has been a steady rise from an average longevity of around 40 years in the late nineteenth century to more than 80 years in some developed countries. This is due largely to declines in infectious diseases which, in turn, have been due not only to the development of antibiotics and other medicines, but also to improvements in public health, sanitation, hygiene and nutrition. It seems clear, then, that economic development (as measured primarily by economic growth) has been 'the single biggest contributor to human health over the last 200 years' and is still needed (although perhaps in a more sustainable form) for today's poor countries.

But while growth and health over the long term appear to be positively related, there is growing evidence to suggest that the situation is more complex in the short term (i.e., 1–10 years). In a range of economies from the US to Japan to Mexico, health indices are negatively affected by economic upturns (booms) and positively affected by downturns (busts). This is also reflected in improvements in health in both the UK and Scandinavia during World War II. More recently, there was a 1000kcal daily average decrease in food intake in Cuba after the Russians withdrew aid in 1989. The country went broke, but there were big improvements in several health indicators. Obesity declined by 50 per cent, heart disease by 35 per cent, stroke by 18 per cent and all-cause mortality by 20 per cent. Nauru, the small Pacific Island country that prospered for 100 years from the export of super-phosphate, had one of the highest rates of obesity and Type 2 diabetes in the world in the 1980s. Since the exhaustion of super-phosphate in the 1990s, there have been dramatic declines in both. In a classic Australian study with Aboriginal men in the early 1980s, Professor Kerin O'Dea, then from the Baker Institute in Melbourne, demonstrated that a return to Indigenous living largely reversed the obesity and diabetes that had developed in the modern Westernised environment.

All this suggests that while there are big improvements in health with growth over the long term, the association is less clear in the short term, with greater short-term improvements in health in years of recession than years of expansion. Although there are no data to prove it, this is unlikely to have happened in the early stages of growth. From a low base, all economic advancement is likely to relate positively to health; it is when growth is mature that problems seem to commence.

This seems to be at odds with the suggestion above that growth has been the single biggest contributor to human health. However, the paradox can be explained by factoring in the dynamic nature of growth and the economic principle of diminishing returns. This simply means that while $1 invested in the early stages of a project may return 10 per cent or 10 cents on the investment, at a later point it becomes 9 per cent, then 8 per cent and so on, until the cost of the investment is more than than the return on this. Researchers from the University of Michigan examined data on economic growth and mortality rates from Sweden over 200 years. The relationship between growth and health, while strongly positive until the first half of the twentieth century, turned moderately negative in the late twentieth century, reflecting a slowdown, or diminishing rate of returns on continuing investment in the growth model. The time period of the tipping points found in Sweden (around the 1970s) also reflects an increase in negative outputs in terms of increased pollution, resource depletion and climate change, suggesting that economic growth beyond a sweet spot can have diminishing and even negative returns on social welfare and health. Although such correlations don't *prove* causality, they do imply that this is the case.

Dr Jose Tapia Granados, a Spanish-American medical doctor with a PhD in economics, has recently attempted to explain the causal pathways linking counter-intuitive economic fluctuations to mortality: why do we seem to be less healthy in economic booms, and more healthy in busts? In booms, he found, the health declines seem to be related to stress, work pressures, lack of sleep, inactivity, social isolation, increased consumption of tobacco, alcohol and saturated fat, traffic injuries and atmospheric pollution, all of which are positively associated with economic prosperity (although some, admittedly, also with economic decline). Increasingly more of these are also being found to be associated with increases in metaflammation, discussed in the previous chapter. In busts, these factors decrease as influences on ill-health, and returns to simpler forms of living appear to result in reductions in chronic disease (and metaflammation).

As is currently being witnessed with booming growth in China and India, the initial stages of improvement in health are associated with a decline in infectious diseases. But beyond a point—the sweet spot in the relationship between human health and economic growth—this is compensated for by a rise in chronic diseases initiated by the social and behavioural factors related to improved economic circumstances, such as easier access to energy-dense foods and energy-saving devices, decreased sleep, increased fiscal pressures and so on. And while longevity continues to increase (albeit at a slower rate), less well-recorded measures, such as the number of years lived with a disability appear to change for the worse, as shown in the rapid rise in obesity in developing countries. While some of this may be simply related to increased ageing, the growth of disability-related disorders such as obesity and Type 2 diabetes at all ages would suggest a maturing population is not the full story.

A potential mediator (although we don't suggest this is the only mediator) is the low-grade systemic form of immune response to chronic disease—metaflammation—discussed in the previous chapter. As we have seen, though, a classical immune response to a bacteria or virus usually results in a restoration of health to normality in the short term. It appears the immune system has not evolved to respond to those changes in behaviours or the environment causing a lesser, but no less dangerous, inflammatory reaction that underlies many modern, lifestyle-related chronic diseases.

Put simply, while the world's population of around 7 billion people espouse to live the life of 300 million Americans, leaving an average carbon footprint of some 24 tonnes of carbon per person per year; while people are encouraged to increase population to facilitate economic growth; while excess consumption of non-renewable resources and processed foods is not only countenanced but demanded by a growth system; and while an estimated average world carbon footprint of around 5 tonnes per person per year with the current population is the 'tipping point' for major climate change, there is little chance of dealing naturally with obesity and/or climate change.

Economists quote a formula for human impact on the environment. This is represented by the IPAT equation, or $I = P \times A \times T$, where I represents the impact on the environment, P is the total population, A is 'affluence' or the income per person, and T is technology. As enlightened as this may sound, the equation has a major flaw: while some economists may finally be taking account of the *ecological* environment in considering the effects of economic growth, they have largely ignored the most important variable to which any economic system should be beholden—human health and wellbeing, or the *biological* environment. As we have seen, health appears to improve dramatically in the early stages of growth, but beyond a certain sweet spot the health returns from further investment in growth appear to decline—at least in the *total* burden of disease.

It may be expected that humans should be able to correct this with the education that comes through economic development (not necessarily the same thing as 'growth'). With education, lifestyles can be changed voluntarily to become healthier, by choosing healthier foods, increasing exercise, not smoking and reducing work-related stress. But while this appears to be intuitively logical, and supported empirically by the obesity flip seen in developing countries when the upper socio-economic classes become leaner as the lower groups become more obese with economic advancement, the reality may not be so simple. The social epidemiologist Sir Michael

Marmot, has shown that the biggest influence on an individual's health is not education, money or social class, but the level of control that person feels she or he has over her or his own life. And while economic growth brings (monetary) wealth, the evidence points to an accompanying *decrease* in feelings of personal control. Also, despite the obesity flip, population levels of obesity continue to increase in just about all countries, despite desperate attempts to insulate populations against this through education. As recently pointed out by Dr Richard Wilkinson, a colleague of Michael Marmot, bigger health problems also occur in countries where the income discrepancy between the upper and lower income earners in a country is greatest, thus leading to less trust and greater feelings of loss of control.

In any case, irrespective of the effects of growth on health, there are undoubted effects on the environment, in the form of increasing pollution, species extinction, severe weather events and climate change. It is to these, and the link between climate change and obesity, to which we will now turn.

CHAPTER 6

LINKING OBESITY, CHRONIC DISEASE AND THE ENVIRONMENT

'. . . increased population adiposity [fatness], because of its contribution to climate change from additional food and transport GHG [greenhouse gases] emissions, should be recognised as an environmental problem'.

PHIL EDWARDS & IAN ROBERTS,
INTERNATIONAL JOURNAL OF EPIDEMIOLOGY

In 2006, the Australian cartoonist Alan Moir published a cartoon in the *Sydney Morning Herald* showing an editorial meeting in a newspaper office. The editor, with a wall poster behind him announcing 'Ultimate Horror Movie Inc' is gesticulating wildly to his staff: 'I see it . . . a story of our times . . . obesity meets global warming!' At the time, the humour lay in the improbability of these two challenging problems being connected. Since then, however, authors, scientists and researchers have shown that this seemingly absurd suggestion has become a frightening reality.

An Australian, Dr Tony McMichael, was innovative in this area: he looked at the potential spread of infectious disease given warming at higher world latitudes. Then Dr Ole Faergeman, a Danish cardiologist, was one of the first to propose a connection with *chronic* disease when he suggested that there are two key issues relating climate change and health: first, diseases caused by climate change (generally infectious diseases reaching higher latitudes because of changed vector breeding conditions as the earth warms up (i.e., as suggested by Dr McMichael)) and secondly, diseases sharing common causes with climate change. And recently, many highly regarded scientific journals—*Obesity Reviews*, the *American Journal of Preventive Medicine*, the *Lancet*, the *British Medical Journal*, the *Medical Journal of Australia* and the *British Journal of Nutrition*—have published articles or editorials linking the causes and potential solutions of obesity and climate change. *New Scientist* even questioned the links with, and benefits of, continued economic growth in this respect. In the UK, two government commissioned reports have linked both problems, stating in one that 'the causes of excess weight are similar to climate change'.

In their book *Globesity*, Francis Delpeuch and colleagues provide a handy diagram of how obesity and greenhouse gas emissions are linked, developed from an earlier German study, and reproduced on the next page as Figure 6.1.

As we've seen, about 15 per cent of the world's population (around 1 billion people) are currently overweight or obese, and this is increasing rapidly with economic growth. The lifestyle changes leading to this and stimulated by such

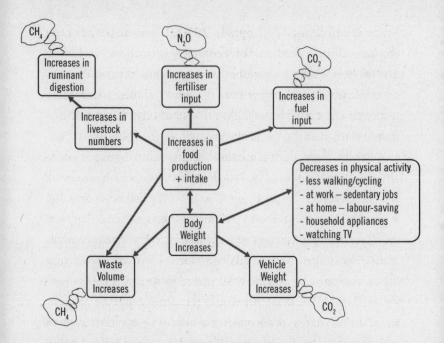

FIGURE 6.1 THE LINK BETWEEN OBESITY AND GREENHOUSE GASES
(from Delpeuch et al., 2009)

growth—beyond the sweet spot—have led also to the rise of a form of metabolic inflammation (metaflammation) in humans in developed countries, associated with a rise in chronic diseases such as Type 2 diabetes, cardiovascular disease, respiratory diseases and certain types of cancers. The types of lifestyle behaviours that have caused this, particularly the overuse of effort-saving technologies and non-renewable fossil fuels in transport, and the over-production and consumption of processed energy-dense foods, are also commonly accepted as contributing to the increases of carbon emissions into the atmosphere from 250 parts per million (ppm) fifty years ago to around 387 ppm in 2010. The increase has been implicated in a number of ecological disorders, including atmospheric pollution, global warming and climate change. So while obesity can contribute to climate change, the factors affecting climate change might also contribute to chronic disease, which previously has been attributed to obesity.

Definite evidence for a causal relationship between obesity and climate change is lacking. But two British scientists have modelled how this might occur. Phil Edwards and Ian Roberts from the London School of Hygiene and Tropical Medicine have estimated the impact of population changes in obesity on greenhouse gas emissions. They calculated that a population with around a 40 per cent obesity level (as predicted for the UK in 2010) would require around 20 per cent more food energy than one with only a 3 per cent rate of obesity (as in 1970). In a world population of 1 billion obese people, extra greenhouse gas emissions are estimated to be between 0.4–1.0 giga tonnes (GT) of carbon dioxide equivalents per year. Given a total global emission of approximately 42 GT of carbon equivalents per year in a world population of 6 billion in 2000, this represents a significant addition to greenhouse gas build-up. Some of this comes from the extra food needed to feed big people, some from the extra energy required to transport them.

Still, while this may provide a description of the link between obesity and climate change, it does little to explain the deeper cause—and hence ways of correcting both situations. To do this requires yet another brief sidetrack, this time into the field of epidemiology.

Epidemiologists are scientists who study the origins and causes of disease. For our purposes, there are two main types: those who study sudden or acute causes of disease, such as an outbreak of bird or swine flu in a country, or an outbreak of food poisoning in an area; and those who study chronic diseases which generally take longer to develop, and are less related to microbial infections.

Acute disease epidemiologists are like detectives who have to work quickly at a scene before the clues are removed. Chronic disease epidemiologists, on the other hand, have comparatively more time. To suggest that a risk factor for heart disease may be a lack of essential marine fats in the diet, based on an observation of the reduced heart disease rate of the Inuit in Greenland, for example, is just the start of decades of trying to prove this through a wide range of different means.

Both types of epidemiologists learn from each other. The strict scientific methodology and statistical rigour required to understand an often unclear association in chronic disease epidemiology can be equally applied to acute diseases to prevent a recurrence once the immediate danger is over, and there is time to reflect. The deductive processes required of acute disease epidemiology, on the other hand, need to be applied by chronic disease epidemiologists to get a full understanding of the different levels of causality of chronic disease. To suggest, for example, that eating too much and not exercising enough causes obesity is like suggesting that the cause of an outbreak of food poisoning is 'a restaurant somewhere'. A good epidemiologist would track the level of causality to its genesis.

In the case of food poisoning, victims would be questioned in order to identify the common factors leading to infection. This might be, for example, a restaurant at, say, 22 Main St, Bongongalong, at which all infected cases were diners on 23 April after 9 p.m. The victims would then be questioned about the food they ate, in order to narrow down the source of infection. This would then be isolated and the reasons for its virulence, such as the type of food preparation, would be ascertained. Only then could the true cause of the outbreak be identified and action taken to stop the disease from spreading (or occurring again). The same deductive processes need to be applied to assessing the true causes of obesity and related chronic disease at the biological level, and climate change at the ecological level.

As discussed in Chapter 2 and illustrated in figure 2.1, external factors, and not just personal sloth and gluttony, can influence energy balance in modern societies and cause obesity and chronic disease. The fact that we now know that obesity is part of a broader inflammatory (metaflammatory) response in the body suggests that the term 'inflammatory environment', may be appropriate for the world we now live in. As well as describing the internal, biological, environment, this also describes the external, or ecological, environment, which is associated with such phenomena as climate change. To do this, though, inflammation needs to be defined a bit more broadly.

According to the *Macquarie Dictionary*, inflammation is 'a disturbance of function following insult or injury'. At the biological level this refers to an immune reaction to correct a disturbance of physiological balance in an individual. At the ecological level it could refer to the disturbance of balance in the broader environment. This is particularly so if we consider the ecosphere as a living, responsive system as proposed by the environmental scientist James Lovelock with his concept of Gaia. In this context, elevated carbon (and other gas) concentrations in the atmosphere resulting from human development constitute an ecological disturbance with symbolic similarities to the metaflammation observed in individuals. This is personified in a statement by Lovelock who says, 'I am a planetary physician whose patient, the living earth, complains of fever.' Increased ocean acidity, atmospheric pollution and global warming are the inflammatory markers that signal such a feverish, abnormal state of the ecosphere, representing 'a disturbance of function following insult or injury', with climate change a metaphorical 'dis-ease' outcome. In 2008, we proposed the term 'ecoflammation' to describe this outcome in line with the metaflammation described earlier.

In this context, if inflammation is a defensive response to a disturbance in the body's status quo, climate change represents a similar response to the disturbance of increased atmospheric pollution, just as lifestyle-related diseases and obesity represent the response to the energy imbalance and other components of our modern lifestyles. The link between biological inflammation (metaflammation) and diseases like Type 2 diabetes and heart disease is not yet totally clear, but it appears that inflammation somehow reduces the ability of insulin produced in the pancreas to transport glucose into the body's cells to be broken down to provide energy. The term used to describe this is insulin resistance. There's plenty of insulin available, but it is inefficient in helping soak up blood glucose. By analogy, the warning sign—the 'insulin resistance'—of the ecosphere is the inability of the planet's sinks (trees, oceans, soil etc.) to soak up excessive carbon emissions, resulting in a form of 'carbon resistance'. Other symptoms of a disturbance of ecological function are 'degradation of land, depletion of resources, accumulation of wastes, pollution of all kinds, climate change, abuses of technology and destruction to biodiversity in all its forms'.

Perhaps surprisingly, the cause (and possible treatment) of both biological and ecological forms of disturbance may not be dissimilar. This is clarified by the epidemiological approach to both problems shown in Figure 6.1, where a similar causal hierarchy is shown between the route to metaflammation, associated with individual biological inflammatory states at the top of the figure, and the ecoflammation, associated with global ecological dis-ease at the bottom.

In a metaphorical sense, we can consider both biological disturbances (diabetes, cardiovascular disease, cancers etc.) and ecological disturbances (storm events, sea level rises, extinctions etc.) shown on the right-hand side of the figure to be forms of 'dis-ease', where this is defined (by the *Macquarie Dictionary*) as 'any deranged or depraved condition'. At the first level of causality there are risk factors and markers that can be identified for both biological and ecological disorders. This is where metaflammation and ecoflammation equate, with insulin resistance and carbon resistance being markers and where the tendency to intervene to correct the situation is usually concentrated.

However, taking the causality further back—let's say to the unclean cooking practices in the food poisoning example—the

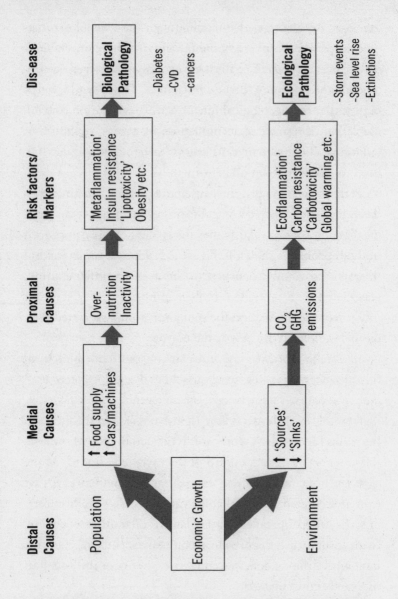

FIGURE 6.2 THE CAUSES OF INFLAMMATION – BIOLOGICAL AND ECOLOGICAL

causes of both forms of inflammatory state begin to merge through the growing misuse of energy: too much energy-dense food consumed in the case of the population and too much fossil fuel burned and waste emissions given off in the case of the broader environment. Both of these, of course, are important current contributors to economic growth. So as well as increasing metaflammation in the individual, too much economic growth has resulted in increasing world levels of atmospheric carbon. The tipping point at which this has been predicted to cause *irreversible* environmental change has been estimated at 450 parts per million (ppm) of carbon, but with a current level of 387 ppm, and increases of 2 ppm per year, growing exponentially, this is likely to be quickly reached.

While we are using metaphor, the spillover concept, as discussed with body fat beyond the sweet spot in Chapter 4, has a similar metaphorical link with carbon emissions into the environment. At a level of sustainability, carbon produced by human and other biological activity is soaked up by sinks in the biosphere. Trees are the best known of these, but plankton, the ocean, the soil, and other components of the geosphere also contribute. However, when carbon emissions into the atmosphere exceed the amount able to be extracted, or soaked up, there is carbon 'spillover', resulting in a build-up of excess carbon—let's call it 'carbotoxicity'—causing ecological disturbances that may be equated with the biological disturbances caused by the toxicity of spillover fat (lipotoxicity) in humans.

Trying to manage carbon emissions, like trying to reduce excess insulin in order to treat diabetes, is a finger in the dyke approach to dealing with the problem. A more global intervention is necessary to deal with the upstream foundation causes shown on the extreme left-hand side of Figure 6.1. This is likely to mean reducing the pressure on the dyke by diverting the stream to a more secure course. It means also stretching our minds to understand the concept of economic growth in the context of human health; how this is fed by both population growth and industrialisation, and why a tipping point will inevitably have to be, and indeed may have already been, reached, for both inflammatory carbon emissions into the atmosphere, to cause serious environmental harm, and metaflammatory reactions in humans, to cause rapid increases in chronic disease.

The challenge of this book has been in trying to relate three major sweet spots in human development—economic growth, body fat and climate change—and the overshooting of these, to the beginnings of economic, population health and environmental problems. For body fat, the sweet spot is relatively easily defined in terms of a mean level of body fat percentage, which gives the minimum prevalence of underweight as well as overweight in the population. The sweet spot for economic growth is the level of GDP at which there are optimal levels of health and wellbeing and a sustainable environment. But things are a little more difficult when talking about a carbon, or environmental, sweet spot.

Environmentally, the world was no doubt better off without (modern) humans, despite the fact that climate changes have obviously occurred throughout time from non-human sources. The point at which balance in the atmosphere was optimal is debatable, because it depends on the, 'optimal for what?' question. The question, however, has become inconsequential for the current discussion. The important point now is that a significant end of the current environmental sweet spot for humans came about when greenhouse gas sources overshot the ability of sinks to soak up their output; when the ecosphere developed what could be termed carbotoxicity, leading to the gradual build-up of atmospheric gases, including carbon, with the ability to raise Gaia from her slumber to provoke a reaction that is likely to be far from sweet—at least for humanity. The sweet spot for the environment, therefore, is at a level of sustainability of environmental resources, including waste gases, habitat and biodiversity, under which sinks exceed sources and equilibrium is maintained.

In summing up, the early stages of economic growth are marked by limited excess consumption and limited availability of pro-inflammatory inducers. They are also marked by huge improvements in human living conditions. (For this reason, some form of 'growth' will be needed in the developing countries for some time to come). Then, as part of advancing growth and increased wealth, there are increases in the consumption of processed energy-dense foods, occupational and personal stress, sleep deprivation and pressures for superfluous consumption (such as smoking and processed fluid intake) to fuel the economic growth system. This is accompanied by a decrease in physical activity due to technological advancement and the availability of energy-saving devices. It is not coincidental that growth begins to yield diminishing returns in human health beyond a point. It is also not coincidental that these changes coincide with major deteriorations in the environment, predisposing to climate change. An epidemio-logical approach to the causes of obesity, and the chronic diseases ascribed to obesity, and of climate change (see Figure 6.1), indicates economic growth is an underlying factor in both. In simple terms, what was once incontrovertibly good for health—economic growth—has begun to display signs of diminishing, or even negative, rates of return, at least in the developed countries.

As an end to exponential growth is inevitable, and as that time is approaching at an accelerating speed (if not already reached), we need next to examine under what circumstances this is likely to occur and how the situation can be optimised. Has our sweet spot in economic growth and human health been surpassed? Do the gathering clouds of financial crisis, over-population, climate change, ecological degradation and even pandemic influenza signal a potential perfect storm, which might not only signal the end of a somewhat obscure sweet spot, but the beginnings of a potential sour spot, which could have serious ramifications for future human wellbeing?

CHAPTER 7

THE PERFECT STORM AND THE SOUR SPOT

'. . . the current optimism is like the man falling from the thirtieth floor of a building who reports "so far so good" when he passes the tenth floor'.

JEFFREY SACHS, *COMMON WEALTH*

In August 1978, the childhood home of one of us (GE), which had existed, untroubled by the elements, for over fifty years on a beachside block on the Central Coast of New South Wales, was washed into the sea over a four-day period. This followed an unprecedented meeting of two major and highly untypical cyclonic fronts less than fifty kilometres off the coast. The impact of this—the shifting of huge rock boulders weighing several tonnes over cliff faces and hundreds of metres of open land—astounded even the most hardened disaster experts. In climatological terms it was described as a one-in-1000-year event.

Such things happen. On 7 February 2009, after a record

tenth day of temperatures above 40 degrees C, the mercury reached 46.7 degrees and winds blew at 130 km/h as a huge fireball swept through the southern Australian state of Victoria, killing almost two hundred people, reducing over 2000 homes to rubble and making more than 7000 people homeless in a period of three to four hours. It was the greatest natural catastrophe in the history of Australia since white settlement. The combination of conditions that created this—a drought, the winds, the vegetation, the extreme temperatures—exemplify the 'perfect storm', just like the cyclones that met to destroy Garry Egger's family home.

A perfect storm (which takes its name from Sebastian Junger's 1997 account of the coming together of two huge weather systems off the Atlantic Coast of North America and the disastrous effect on stranded fishing fleets), is a special type of experience—a sour spot, if you like. It's a time when the gods are frowning, and when a range of nasty events that *can* come together to make a catastrophe *do* come together. Usually, as with a sweet spot, there is a build-up to a sour spot, through a number of factors propitiating the perfect storm. Clouds start to gather, events occur and processes are initiated, all of which lead to a force greater than the sum of its parts with an outcome which is immediately negative from the majority perspective. Take, for example, the events that led to the outbreak of World War II in Europe. It all began with the establishment of the Weimar Republic following German discontent with the Treaty of Versailles, the advent of the Great Depression with its high rates of disaffected unemployed people in 1930, an enfeebled West, and the rising aspirations of Adolf Hitler.

At a more personal level, a sour spot in a family or relationship can come from months or years of events that build to a crescendo: an outbreak of violence, an unbridgeable communication gap or the chance meeting of a new partner that signifies the apex (or perhaps nadir) of the perfect storm.

While the outcome of a sweet spot is happiness, contentment or bliss, the outcome of a sour spot is catastrophe. Its extreme is death: for the individual, the family, the population or parts of the biosphere. It is not uncommon for a perfect storm, or sour spot, to follow a sweet spot, or for a sweet spot to follow a perfect storm. Indeed, if this were not the case, life would be pretty dull. In between, there are zones which we could call the 'okay zone' and the 'not okay zone'. In the former, things are going along okay, as the name suggests, but not perfectly, as in a sweet spot, or disastrously, as in a sour spot. In the not okay zone, things are not so good, but could get better, even to the point of a sudden and unexpected sweet spot, or worse, to the extent of a gradually developing sour spot. Shifts between the okay and not okay zones are also common, and unexpected jumps from an okay period to a sour spot—as in a sudden accident—or from a not okay period to a sweet spot—as in a sudden windfall—happen frequently.

Most sweet spots and sour spots are localised, if not to a small geographical area then to a limited number of people or conditions they influence. But depending on the situation, they can be more general, even to the level of a national triumph or disaster. The United States appeared to hit a sweet spot as a nation around the end of World War II when soldiers returned home to a high level of optimism and promising living conditions. An Iraqi sour spot came at the end of a perfect storm of American hegemony and Saddam Hussein's arrogance, culminating in the 'Shock and Awe' invasion of 2003.

Throughout history, a limited number of sweet or sour spots have engaged the entire world. The industrial revolution of the nineteenth century and both major wars of the twentieth century are examples. In a sweeping analysis, the Cambridge historian Nicholas Boyle has claimed that great events—some sweet, some sour, some mixed—have marked the middle of the second decade of each new century for the last five hundred years. For example:

- In 1517, Martin Luther published his thesis which started the Reformation, the beginning of a long sweet or sour spot (depending on one's orientation) dictating world theology;
- In 1618 the Thirty-Year War began in Europe, ushering in a century of religious conflict;
- In 1715 the death of Louis XIV in France, following the settlement of the war of the Spanish succession and the accession of the Hanoverians in Britain in 1714, marked a sweet spot of peaceful trade and the development of democracies across Europe;
- In 1815 the Napoleonic era ended with Bonaparte's defeat at Waterloo, and a long British sweet spot based on trade began, together with a relatively peaceful period throughout Europe;
- In 1914, World War I commenced and a succession of rolling sour spots began, concluding only at the end of World War II in 1945.

Although admitting this analysis is somewhat tongue-in-cheek, Boyle suggests a possible causative association for a build-up of events like this: an inter-generational change, where those who come into power around the turn of each century think of that century as their own, in contrast to the previous one of their antecedent generation.

The coming together of a variety of factors at the end of the first decade of the third millennium, together with the beginnings of negative returns on the growth model of economics, signalled yet another early-century epochal event, the nature of which is not yet clear. It could be a catastrophic sour spot, as in 1914, which could undermine a way of life which people in advanced countries have come to unconsciously think is a natural right of human progress. Alternatively, it could be the beginning of a peaceful sweet spot of co-operation as began in 1815: a new way of thinking, a new world revolution, following the agrarian and industrial revolutions of the 1700s.

What are the factors that have led us to this point? Apart from those discussed to date—the coming end of the current model of growth, climate change, and an obesity epidemic—there are at least four of which the public has become increasingly aware. In the first place we have just (at least for the moment) overcome a global economic crisis the likes of which the world has never seen, which, if looked at broadly, requires not just a stimulation of the existing economic system but a change in the growth paradigm which has driven the world over the last two centuries. Secondly, we have a world population which has risen exponentially from around 1 billion in 1800 to around 2 billion in 1900 to a predicted 9 billion by 2050, reminiscent of the level of lemmings, or field mice in a good season, before a predicted Malthusian collapse. Thirdly, there is the rise in pollution and human waste which threatens to overwhelm the biosphere's sinks leading to climate change. Fourthly, resources, organisms and species are disappearing at a rate never before experienced, creating 'feedback' if one believes the self-regulating earth philosophy (Gaia) of James Lovelock, that will worsen all the other factors mentioned.

There is yet another factor, which this book has concentrated on, which puts into focus the human side of all of the above. This is the subtle change in human health now beginning to appear in developed countries. Obesity is the signal of this change. For a while we continue to live *longer* in the presence of rising obesity rates. Kept alive by access to plentiful food, sophisticated public health systems, advanced knowledge of hygiene and the marvels of modern medicine, there is a rising tide of chronic diseases (for which obesity is the beacon), making us question whether we are living *better* today than in previous times. Add to this the long-expected threat of an infectious disease outbreak to rival the great influenza pandemic of 1918–19, and we have a not okay build-up to a perfect storm. The swine flu outbreak of 2009, although less virulent in its early stages than was originally predicted, could well be the forerunner for a deadly viral mutation which could capitalise on the converging conditions of a potential worldwide perfect storm. The question that remains is what do we need to do to ensure the world moves towards a sweet spot and away from a potential sour spot. Some answers are suggested in the remaining chapters of this book.

CHAPTER 8

HEALTH PROMOTION FOR ECONOMISTS

'All we have to do to destroy the planet's climate and
biota and leave a ruined world to our children and
grandchildren is to keep doing exactly what we are doing
today, with no growth in the human population or the
world economy.'

JAMES GUSTAVE SPETH,
THE BRIDGE AT THE EDGE OF THE WORLD

As we have seen, the economic system under which the
world currently operates is like a freight train gathering
speed while heading for a cliff. To make things worse, the
drivers have their heads in the engine room stoking the fire,
and are unwilling or unable to look up to see where the train
is heading.

A much discussed alternative is the steady state economy—
that is, an economy in which the throughputs are sustainable

over an infinite period. As well as being suggested by the great early economic architects, such as John Stuart Mill, J.M. Keynes and even Adam Smith, the grandfather of capitalism, it appears logical that, in some form, a steady state economy must be the eventual outcome of the growth system. It is only necessary to consider the nature of any exponential system. Thus, one dollar invested at the time of Jesus Christ at a 5 per cent interest rate, if placed in a pile, would now reach as far as the stratosphere.

Under the current growth system, world economic activity (which involves the exponential use of limited natural resources), has increased six-fold in the last thirty years. With an expected 9 billion people on the planet by 2050, all aspiring to the affluence the OECD countries enjoy today, a further fifteen-fold increase in the economy would be needed, and a forty-fold increase by the end of the century. As current resource use and waste development is already at or near its limits (as indicated by climate change), this is clearly not sustainable.

One approach to the dilemma of growth is to call for decoupling of the notion of progress from material through-put and consumption. There are two forms of decoupling: relative and absolute. Relative decoupling basically means doing more with less so that renewable resources begin to replace non-renewable ones, thus slowing the rate of environmental impact. (Technically, resource impacts decline relative to GDP. The impacts may still increase, but they do so more slowly than GDP.) Absolute decoupling occurs when only renewable resources are used and there is also reduced per capita consumption. (Technically, there is no increase in impacts but unlimited increases in GDP.) Economists often talk of decoupling as if it will happen naturally without breaching ecological limits. But probably the best we can hope for, at least in the immediate future, is a relative decoupling. However, with increasing population growth, even this is unlikely as absolute resource depletion is increased. The concept of sustainable growth based on absolute decoupling, while an attractive alternative, is highly unlikely in the current political climate. Meantime, while the link between growth and climate change is vigorously debated, the health sciences are conspicuously under-represented, particularly in relation to the relevance of economic growth to the world obesity and chronic disease epidemics.

A steady state economy, in some form, has to be the minimum long-term goal. (Some ecological economists, such as Serge Latouche from the University of Paris-Sud, believe a 'de-growth' society is our only long-term alternative, given that the earth's resources and natural cycles cannot sustain the economic growth which is the essence of capitalism and modernity.) But shifting to a steady state economy will clearly involve a major disruption to business as usual, and will not come rapidly or without pain. The difficulty lies in getting traditional economists involved in lateral thinking. As pointed out by the science philosopher Thomas Kuhn, paradigm shifts in science, which are the way in which knowledge advances, involve stages of denial, ridicule, resistance and opposition before any hint of interest and acceptance. This was probably put best by the great Indian liberator Mahatma Gandhi in his comment on social change: 'First they ignore you. Then they laugh at you. Then they fight you. Then you win.'

In the first instance it would help to redefine the current measure of economic success: GDP. As a measure of throughput, it is clearly at odds with optimising human health. As J. Eric Oliver, author of *Fat Politics* points out: '. . . most of our basic necessities have long ago been met and our worker productivity is so great, economic growth can only be sustained through greater consumption, that is by convincing Americans to buy more than their essential needs.'

The illth (i.e., products with monetary value but potential unhealthy impact) created in monetary terms is posted as progress when measuring GDP. A better measure of progress, which includes human health and wellbeing, must be considered. While several of these have been mooted—for example gross domestic happiness or well-being indexes—they have yet to be debated or taken seriously by traditional economists and politicians. A possible reason is the modern divergence between the generally acknowledged benefits of economic development and the monetary figure used to measure economic growth. An end to the latter would suggest to most economists and politicians an end to the former. However, according to John Stuart Mill:

'. . . a stationary condition of capital and population implies no stationary state of human improvement. There would be as much scope as ever for all kinds of mental culture, and moral and social progress; as much and much more likelihood of it being improved, when minds cease to be engrossed by the art of getting on.'

A more modest ambition before a shift to a more complete measure of progress or a steady state system would be an open debate about the relative advantages of an alternative economic system. Currently, those with vested but short-sighted interest in maintaining the status quo, including the media, stifle this. Eloquent spokespersons like Clive Hamilton and Ian Lowe in Australia, while highly respected in limited circles, are given little opportunity in the open media. In the health arena, such contributors are notable by their absence in the climate or environmental debate. In the UK the Sustainable Development Commission (SDC) is a considerable step in the right direction, particularly as its March 2009 report, 'Prosperity without Growth', discusses the alternatives to the current growth system, but within a progress (development) paradigm. The report concludes with a recommendation of three main tasks for government (see note 3):

1. to develop and apply a robust macro-economics for sustainability;
2. to redress the damaging and unsustainable social logic of consumerism;
3. to establish and impose meaningful resource and environmental limits on economic activity. [Human health could possibly be added here.]

Consumerism, while fuelling the current economic growth model, receives considerable attention from the SDC, but is often not considered at all in other discussions of economic exchange. Indeed the association between increased consumption and increased living standards is seemingly locked in to the Western (and now the developing world's) psyche. Correction to this way of thinking will require significant shifts in community attitudes, some of which, surprisingly, may occur spontaneously, but much of which will need direction through legislation initiating behavioural change. The role of personal carbon trading as one way of doing this is discussed in the next chapter.

The second big issue to resolve is population growth. At first glance this may appear irrelevant. Population can be clearly linked with carbon emissions and climate change—but obesity, and chronic disease? Surely population growth, through expanding financial resources, ensures the advances in medicine that can help reduce the incidence of disease?

It is hoped that by now the falsity of this connection can be seen. Economic growth is traditionally driven by three main factors: resource discovery, technological change and population growth. As we know, accessible, non-renewable resources are becoming rapidly depleted, so they cannot continue to drive economic growth in the long term. Certainly there is pressure on technological development to lead consumerism, but population growth is presently the easiest, most politically acceptable way to encourage economic growth, particularly as reproduction is a biological imperative. All round the world, governments have cemented power in recent years through promises of population expansion, baby bonuses, and baby smooching at election time. They also promise increased immigration to fill low-paying jobs, overcome skills shortages and to increase economic growth. But has this familiar litany now passed its used-by date?

The projected 50 per cent addition to our world population by 2050 would mean that just to maintain the 2009 status quo in relation to carbon emissions there would need to be a very significant level of decoupling between growth and resource use. In a country like Australia, with a current population of around 20 million (actually ~23 million) people presently responsible for emissions of 25 tonnes of carbon per person per year, a rise to a population of 30 million people would mean a 50 per cent reduction in carbon production on this basal rate would be needed just to stay level—and even this is well above the estimated 4–5 tonnes pp/py estimated as a world average requirement just to maintain stability. As undeveloped countries, at a current level of around 2–4 tonnes pp/py strive to reach the lifestyle that matches the US level of 24 tonnes pp/py, the sustainable level becomes a moving target ever harder to achieve.

A common argument against planned population control is that the biggest influence on female fecundity is education. Hence, increased economic growth, which usually implies increased education, should have an automatic effect of slowing population growth. But the same economic growth that accompanies declining birth rates *increases* the carbon footprint of each individual, resulting in a greater total environmental impact, even with a smaller population. Also, as seen in Australia, birth rates can be raised instantaneously on a government whim, by providing incentives such as the baby bonus introduced by John Howard during his third term in office, irrespective of the overall education level of the population. Then, the Australian birth rate rose from 1.7 to 1.9 children per female within two years. (The generally successful one-child policy of China, the world's biggest country, while not likely to be condoned in a democratic society, shows that government policy can also have a dampening effect on birth rates.)

The tragedy about the population debate is that it is hindered by the politics of timidity. Groups like the World Wildlife Fund, Greenpeace and other conservation groups are afraid of losing their constituency among families with more than two children (i.e., higher than replacement value) if they raise the issue. The fact that is ignored, however, by those with large families who take discussion of that issue as a personal slight, is that this is not about the past, it is about the future. Large families in the past were necessary to get the human race to its developmental sweet spot, because of high infant and early adult mortality. But the life of all species is dynamic and has to adapt to both natural and unnatural change, not just to thrive, but to survive.

So as population increases are the simplest way to promote economic growth, as economic growth is dependent on consumption, and as consumption (at least in its present form) includes eating more and moving less, there is a perverse link between population growth and obesity. Purchasing and using a large, gas-guzzling vehicle has been a patriotic act in growth-dominated economies like the US, as this contributes significantly to consumption and thus to growth. A shift to renewable fuel, if and when this happens, could help decouple the economy, but would do little for obesity. Also, because of the energy costs and resource use of vehicle production, the increasing numbers of vehicles required to service a growing population and hence re-stimulate the economy would serve to *re*-couple any decoupling of the economy that may have occurred through a shift to renewable fuels.

A solution to this, of course, would be personal responsibility, where individual consumers purchase only goods and services that would reduce energy intake or increase energy expenditure—for example, weight loss programs and operations, exercise machines, gym equipment and bicycles for transport—and, in the process, possibly reduce their carbon footprint. As many individuals in industrial societies manage to stay lean, it can obviously be done. However, as any social behaviour expert knows, appeals to personal responsibility—in opposition to hedonism and personal gratification—generally fall short. This is evidenced by the fact that following significant increases in knowledge about healthy behaviours through health promotion campaigns, adherence to a healthy lifestyle pattern actually decreased in the US in the eighteen years from 1988 to 2006. Concurrently, there was a rise in obesity in half of the fifty US states and no fall in the number of obese people in any state. It seems the economic pressures to consume overwhelm any biological pressures to live healthily (in the US, at any rate).

Meanwhile, there are smaller but no less significant sacred cows than economic and population growth to be herded in if obesity and climate change are to be contained. Harvard University Forestry Professor and environmentalist James Gustave Speth examines a number of these anomalies—and possible solutions—within the current political and business systems in his environmental critique *The Bridge at the Edge of the World*.

First, Speth contends that private funding of election campaigns makes a mockery of any hint of impartial democracy in political decisions that relate to corporate profit-making, much of which concerns the sale and consumption of fattening and carbon-emitting product. The political power of the food industry, as just one example, is legendary in limiting the concerns of health specialists. When a 2002 Australian government report, commissioned to recommend the biggest bang for the buck in obesity interventions, came up with statistical evidence for restricting junk food advertising to children as the number one priority, the report was shelved, never to see the light of day. Instead, innocuous initiatives with little chance of offending corporate supporters, such as 'promoting physical activity', were released as more politically expedient (see also Chapter 10). In a similar fashion, carbon trading momentum staggers between stalled and reverse.

The second imperative signalled by Speth is elimination of the concept of limited liability in corporate law. The financial crisis of 2008–9 saw billionaire executives walking away from bankrupted corporations with their fortunes intact and no personal responsibility for the millions of lives affected. Yet more than two hundred years ago, Adam Smith, the father of capitalism, recognised that 'managers of other people's money . . . cannot be well expected [to] watch over it with the same anxious vigilance they would their own money'. Corporate shareholders, too, are culpable. Normally reasonable, considered and moral individuals, under the guise of anonymity and driven by profit, they can become as avaricious as any marauding pack of locusts foraging a paddock. And while ethical investment options can be a salve for an investor's conscience, they are often about as realistic as sensitive investment bankers! Similarly, the sale of carbon offsets that require forty years to mature and may have long-term counter-productivity should be open to greater scrutiny. The removal of limited liability (which, like financial deregulation, was originally designed to open up growth in the face of natural declines), would make corporations and their shareholders more conscious of their global environmental and personal health impacts. Of course this would also need to be accompanied by the banning of facile legislation like the Personal Responsibility in Food Consumption Act (aka the 'Cheeseburger Bill') introduced into the US Congress in 2004, following an attempted legal action against restaurants and food-makers for their role in promoting obesity.

A third, apparently unrelated, but highly pertinent problem pointed out by Speth is the externalisation of costs by corporations. This means that factors such as pollution, ill-health, obesity and other adverse effects caused to individuals by corporations in their pursuit of profits are regarded as 'literally, other people's problems. Only pragmatic concern for its own interests and the laws of the land constrain the corporation's predatory instincts, and often that is not enough to stop it from destroying lives, damaging communities, and endangering *the planet as a whole.*' Addition of the costs of externalities to a corporate bottom line would no doubt help in the fight against both obesity and climate change. While there are currently environmental impact statements required for new projects with a potential to damage the environment, no such 'health impact' requirements are necessary for new products or services that may influence or damage human health.

While the suggestions made here go nowhere near solving the joint problems of chronic disease and climate change, they offer an insight into the types of structural change that are usually overlooked in discussions of the former, if not the latter. This is important because, in the words of the Sustainable Development Commission: 'Urging people to act on CO_2, to insulate their homes, turn down their thermostat, put on a jumper, drive a little less, walk a little more, holiday at home, buy locally produced goods (and so on) will either go unheard or be rejected as manipulation for as long as all the messages about high street consumption point in the opposite direction.'

According to the Commission, there are two kinds of structural change that are necessary: 'The first will be to dismantle or correct the perverse incentives for unsustainable (and unproductive) status competition. The second must be to establish new structures that provide capabilities for people to flourish, and particularly to participate fully in the life of society, in less materialistic ways.'

A further conundrum that needs to be considered by the genuinely concerned is whether to do essentially nothing and instead pursue a 'business as usual' approach in order to expedite the problems which will only resonate with voters and their political masters once they have surpassed a threshold of seriousness. This may not be as inconsiderate as it seems at first blush. In talking about restraining population growth, the Australian writer Mark O'Connor considers the public-spirited exhortation to 'save water': '. . . any water restraint shown by an individual citizen will only allow our politicians to persist longer in their folly [of population growth], and will lead—quite soon—to even worse shortages of water, plus many other environmental disasters.'

Similarly, in terms of climate change and obesity reduction, reduced consumption by concerned individuals would only have the effect of delaying the acceptance of the need for structural change by politicians and voters. According to the authors of *Globesity*: 'The politicians will probably be obliged to hold off until our system of production and consumption has become so thoroughly untenable, so absurdly wasteful and its health costs such an unsustainable burden on the community, that the urgent need to do something about it will be glaringly obvious to all.'

A possible alternative to improve health and avoid this philosophically unpalatable solution would be to promote stealth interventions, whereby change is initiated without the public being aware of it having health implications. For example, a stealth intervention for obesity would be one done for another purpose that has a side-effect of more physical activity and/or less energy intake. It is to this, and to individual ways of coping with the environmental influences on health and climate change, to which we will now turn.

CHAPTER 9
MAKING CORRECTIONS

'Governments care about health provision. And the recent focus on wellbeing has extended that concern to psychological health. At the same time, these goals too often take second place to economic growth.'

TIM JACKSON, *PROSPERITY WITHOUT GROWTH*

The discussion so far has been based around a number of assertions, namely that:

- Obesity is rapidly increasing worldwide;
- This may be a signal of deeper underlying causes of chronic disease;
- Chronic disease, obesity and climate change all have the same root cause: economic growth beyond the sweet spot;
- Dealing independently with chronic disease, obesity and climate change may only have a partial, and possibly palliative, effect;

- Major structural changes, particularly in the economic system, but also to the factors which affect it, such as population growth, attitudes to consumption and the behaviour of corporations, are necessary to reduce chronic disease, obesity and climate change.

Some suggestions have been made in the previous chapter for structural change, which usually comes only slowly and against powerful opposition. However, the economic crisis of 2008–9 presents a unique opportunity for change. As pointed out by the conservative economist Milton Friedman: 'Only a crisis—actual or perceived—produces real change. When that crisis occurs, the actions that are taken depend on the ideas that are lying around.' The report of the Sustainable Development Commission, quoted in the previous chapter, is one of the boldest and most practical working documents yet produced for dealing with environmental, economic and personal sustainability issues. This proposes twelve steps under three main policy areas, as follows.

A. Building a Sustainable Macro-economy
   1. Developing macro-economic capability
   2. Investing in jobs, assets and infrastructure
   3. Increasing financial and fiscal prudence
   4. Improving macro-economic accounting

B. Protecting capabilities for flourishing
   5. Sharing the work and improving the work–life balance
   6. Tackling systemic inequalities

7. Measuring prosperity
8. Strengthening human and social capital
9. Reversing the culture of consumerism

C. Respecting ecological limits
10. Imposing clearly defined resource and emission caps
11. Fiscal reform for sustainability
12. Promoting technology transfer and ecosystem protection.

Several of the steps are currently being developed in different disciplinary areas. However, there has so far been limited consideration, within the current research, given to initiatives aimed specifically at improving human health; for example, by decreasing obesity and chronic disease. Carbon trading is a possible exception. Corporate carbon trading (CCT), which has been most widely considered, is designed to reduce carbon energy expenditure at the point of production. As well as reducing total carbon emissions and therefore having a potential impact on climate change, this could conceivably have an effect on the price of processed (and usually high energy-dense) foods, comparative to non-processed (and usually low energy dense) foods. CCT is currently under consideration by many governments, and depending on the outcome of intense political lobbying is likely to come into practice worldwide in some form in the future. Unfortunately, there is currently little involvement by health experts in CCT planning, which could represent a major missed opportunity.

Less well known than CCT is a proposal for personal carbon trading (PCT) initially published in the UK in 1996. This has significant potential for reduction of both obesity (and chronic disease) and climate change. How would it work? Well, carbon emissions from the oxidation of organic fuel sources make up around 80 per cent of the world's greenhouse gases. These can now be accurately measured and attributed to specific quantities of energy use; for example, per unit of fuel, electricity, heating, cooling, etc. (see Table 9.1). Individual carbon emissions, and hence energy use, are thus able to be given a value that could be traded on an open market like any other commodity.

TABLE 9.1 GLOBAL WARMING POTENTIAL OF GASES RELEASED FROM COMBUSTION OF FUELS

Fuel	Carbon units
Human energy	—
Natural gas	0.2 per kilowatt hours
Grid electricity (night)	0.6 per kilowatt hours
Grid electricity (day)	0.7 per kilowatt hours
Petrol	2.3 per litre
Diesel	2.4 per litre
Coal	2.9 per litre
(1 kg of carbon dioxide = 1 carbon unit)	

The concept of individual carbon trading, first proposed by Aubrey Meyer of the Global Commons Institute in the United Kingdom in 1996, stimulated interest in the development of a workable financial incentive system that would provide equity and efficiency in reducing non-renewable energy use and greenhouse gas emissions. A system of contraction and convergence was suggested, with annual contraction of global carbon emissions over a number of years to an agreed sustainable, safe level, and convergence towards equal per capita emissions globally through trade of emission rights between frugal energy users (usually the poor) and profligate emitters (usually the rich).

An individual carbon trading system would overcome the huge deficiencies of current carbon offset systems, whereby trees are planted in the hope that they will soak up atmospheric carbon. Known by a number of names, perhaps the most current of which is Tradable Energy Quotas, the scheme is based on the premise that 40–50 per cent of all energy use occurs at the individual and household levels. Hence, while a corporate cap and trade system for carbon emissions (now accepted by most governments) may help reduce greenhouse gases, if the demand for energy among consumers remains high, the marketplace will overcome price rises.

In a personal carbon trading scheme, the plan is to allocate every individual an equal number of tradable energy units per year, based on 40–50 per cent of a total budget (that includes both personal and corporate quotas) set by a central budgetary council, or carbon bank. Each unit is equivalent to 1 kg of carbon released through energy usage. Trade of units is conducted either through existing credit cards or through a carbon card system administered by banks, and units are redeemed when paying for non-renewable energy (mainly fuel and power).

Individuals who are left with carbon credits (i.e., those who are frugal with non-renewable energy use) are then able to sell these back into the marketplace, thereby gaining financial benefit. Those who overuse their quota pay a premium price for extra energy use. Allocated and tradable carbon allowances would be set by an independent carbon bank managed through current market systems, would be equitable, allow flexible goals to be set into the future and would provide a possible stealth intervention for decreasing metaflammatory states, including obesity. Such a scheme, although requiring considerable political and public will (and unlikely to be unchallenged by vested interests), would be relatively easy to administer once accepted.

A personal carbon trading scheme is equitable as convergence occurs within countries from rich, high-energy users to poor, frugal users, and between countries, also from rich to poor, serving as a more empowering alternative to aid. Unused units are retired, with a view to contraction of the total energy budget to a sustainable level of around 5 tonnes of carbon pp/py.

As a personal carbon trading system would reduce energy use and therefore carbon emissions, the potential effects on climate change should be obvious. The impact on obesity and chronic disease, on the other hand, is perhaps at first a little less apparent, yet the proposed effects shown in Table 9.2 are readily achievable. With more incentive to use person power instead of machines, more energy would be expended and more body fat burned. Even the reduced use of air-conditioning could have an impact, as this has been suggested as another possible contributor to weight gain.

Possibly more important, though, would be the change in attitudes to extravagant energy use a personal trading scheme would cause, where the lust for non-renewable (and often fattening) consumables would be reduced and the importance of health elevated through a form of stealth intervention. Although attitudes are usually thought to be determinants of behaviour, it often occurs the other way around: attitudes can be changed as a result of behaviour change initiated through legislative action. Random breath testing, seatbelt usage and pool safety are all examples of attitudes following behaviour that has been legislated or regulated. The dictum 'legislate and regulate where you can; educate and motivate where you can't' is thus a good principle for health promotion.

For personal carbon trading, a desired long-term outcome would be a shift in consumer aspirations from conspicuous consumption to conspicuous non-consumption; the importance of health would be elevated almost coincidentally. As suggested by the former UK Chief Scientist Sir David King, when asked by a young woman what she could do personally to prevent climate change: 'Stop admiring young men who drive Ferraris.'

The PCT proposal is not meant as a panacea or a single-step approach to either obesity or climate change. Nor is it likely to be as easy to effect as it might seem here. Political will and public acceptance are obviously major factors which need to be carefully considered. Other issues, including concessions, for example through national tax systems, would also need to be looked at within countries, e.g. for those in essential industries and in remote areas. Finally it will be necessary to overcome the small but vociferous band of deniers, not just of climate change but even the epidemic of obesity.

TABLE 9. 2 POTENTIAL EFFECTS OF PERSONAL CARBON TRADING ON INDIVIDUAL HEALTH AND THE BROADER ENVIRONMENT

Potential impacts of PCT on obesity and health

- Conspicuous moderate or non-consumption becomes acceptable in contrast to over-consumption
- Personal energy use for transport (e.g., walking, cycling) is increased
- Changed attitudes to car and active transport use
- Infrastructure for personal energy use (walking, cycling etc.) is more valued, encouraging greater personal energy use
- Shift from cars to active transport

Potential impacts of PCT on the environment

- Personal carbon quotas lead to frugality of use of non-renewable energy
- Reduction of carbon emissions into the atmosphere. Reduced climate change
- Desire for better energy efficiency and development of renewable energy
- Reduced air pollution; improved energy efficiency; altered town planning to increase emphasis on personal mobility
- Changed attitude to consumption; rise of conspicuous frugality
- Greater appreciation and demand for renewable energy
- Reduced car and coal gas (electricity) pollution
- Reduced demand on energy supplies leading to less likelihood of outages in peak periods
- Demand for improved architecture in homes, hotels etc. Increased importance of renewable heating, cooling sources
- Demand for improved energy efficiency of appliances and heating/cooling systems
- Increased demand for low energy-dense, locally grown, unprocessed food products, reducing food transport

Through reduction in non-renewable energy sources and less pressure on sinks, a more sustainable economic and ecological system is encouraged

Other authors have dealt with deniers of climate change extensively. George Monbiot, for example, shows that deniers generally have a vested interest underpinning their stance, usually financial. Thus the large energy companies, likely to lose under carbon trading, are frequently deniers, just as cigarette manufacturers sought to debunk the link between smoking and lung disease from the 1950s through to the 1990s. However, recent technological developments, particularly the internet, have led to the resurgence of another type of denier: the conspiracy theorist denier. This is usually an average, and sometimes highly intelligent, individual with little comprehensive understanding of the different levels of evidence required to reach a scientific conclusion. Couple that with access to the worldwide web, and you have one very self-empowered (albeit misguided) individual. The worldwide web is a publishable source for any would-be spokesperson for any cause, without restriction. It can be picked up by anyone and quoted as fact, and then passed on to others in a form of Chinese Whispers. The instance of the prominent botanist David Bellamy quoting a web-page by a writer much less qualified than himself is a good example within Bellamy's high-profile, but discredited, stance against climate change.

But before coming down too heavily on those with an alternative view, perhaps it's best to let communication principles play themselves out. A long-held health promotion principle called counter-argument occurs when people are forced into one decision or its opposite as a result of being presented two opposing views, one of which is obviously lacking in substance.

For example, one of the first community quit smoking campaigns in the world was conducted by the NSW Health

Department in the 1970s. It was attacked by an elderly smoking doctor–lawyer representing cigarette company interests, Dr William Whitby. Whitby claimed that not only is smoking not dangerous, it's actually good for you! Initially, health officials were concerned as Dr Whitby had compliant support from a media still indebted to cigarette advertising. The officials soon became aware, though, that every time the good doctor appeared to rebut the health facts presented to the community of the North Coast of NSW, the quit program was overwhelmed with demand from smokers wanting to quit. So counter-argument on climate change, as well as on the true causes of obesity, is likely to hasten the demand for a decision, one way or the other, among the general public. And it is only this which is likely to have an impact on politicians and policy-makers. Provided the media is balanced (and that's not guaranteed), the outcome is likely to be positive all round.

In the meantime, the question is what can governments do, and what can we do for ourselves, to reduce both climate change and obesity in our own backyards?

CHAPTER 10
JUST HELP YOURSELF

'As you get more of anything, each addition to what you have—whether loaves of bread or cars—contributes less to your well-being. If you are hungry, a loaf of bread is everything but when your hunger is satisfied, many more loaves don't help you and might become a nuisance as they go stale.'

WILKINSON R., PICKETT K., '*THE SPIRIT LEVEL*'

A major premise of our argument to this point has been that increasing obesity levels in the population are as much a sign of problems in the environment as they are of ill-health in the individual. They are the 'canary in the coalmine' warning us of bigger problems in the environment. Of even more significance to the rising rates of chronic disease in industrialised societies are modern lifestyles driven by an economic system that seems to have passed its sweet spot.

While some of the lifestyle and environmental factors

contributing to chronic disease may contribute to obesity—inactivity, over-eating—others (such as smoking, depression, inadequate sleep and pollution) can have the same health outcome without weight gain, through a form of metaflammation in the body. Simultaneously, some of these factors can also cause 'ecoflammation' in the environment. Given this scenario, individual weight loss may not be vital to the reduction of chronic disease. Instead, this will need to be achieved by bigger structural changes in the environment.

A number of questions arise from this. First, should we be bothering to develop public health initiatives in obesity prevention and encouraging weight loss in individuals? Is this just a cosmetic problem in which governments and clinicians do not need to get involved? Secondly, are current government initiatives likely to have any effect anyway? And finally, what can be done personally to reduce one's risk of chronic disease, help mitigate climate change and maintain a desirable weight in the process?

In response to the first question—whether obesity prevention is important—there is still a need for weight loss and obesity prevention initiatives. This is because, as we have seen, a portion of chronic disease is related to excess body fat in some form. It is safest for everyone to stay within a recommended body weight level. Furthermore, extra weight gain, even in those for whom weight does not currently seem to pose health risks, could ultimately increase such risks when it gets to the level of spillover, or results in psychological or orthopaedic problems.

So while weight loss alone, without other changes in lifestyle and/or the environment (if this were possible), may not have a huge impact on chronic disease levels (despite the current recommendations of several medical groups), there will be some lowering of the incidence of disease, possibly due to reductions in spillover fat. If by unlikely chance some magic pill was discovered which caused weight loss without the need to alter behaviour, this would not drastically reduce chronic disease, as inactivity, poor nutrition, stress, depression, smoking and poor sleep are all independent risk factors for disease, irrespective of body weight. This has been shown clearly in a number of longitudinal studies throughout the world. In general, the progression to Type 2 diabetes in people at high risk is least in those who comply with the most lifestyle changes, including and additional to weight loss. Weight loss remains important in disease management, however, because the correct strategies include changes to the lifestyle causes discussed here, and such changes are likely to have a positive effect on metaflammation, as well as body weight.

So weight loss initiatives and programs at the public health and individual levels, apart from the structural changes needed to have a major impact, are still important. The next question is, do any of them work? And if so, which ones?

In June 2009, an Australian Joint Party report, 'Weighing it Up', was tabled in the Commonwealth parliament. Australia had led the world in recognising population increases in obesity as an issue, with the world's first nationally commissioned report, 'Acting on Australia's Weight', published in 1997. But that report's hundred or so recommendations were largely ignored (with the exception of the development of National Clinical Guidelines in Obesity Management and National Guidelines in Physical Activity). Several reports and committees on obesity followed, all to large media fanfare, but many committees were disbanded before even reporting, and others' recommendations went unheeded.

As a witness before the 'Weighing it Up' Committee, one of us (GE) was told privately by a member that while the 'obesogenic' environment (i.e., one that encourages the development of obesity) argument had merit, this could not seriously be considered by government because it would be against the interests of parliamentary committee members with farmers among their constituents. There is little doubt there were other 'experts' whose evidence was also categorically negated. The innocuousness of the consequent report and government enquiries should be seen for what they are: highly publicised efforts to be seen to be doing something, while keeping the economic train on the tracks by not really doing anything.

This is not meant to be a criticism of any one government, or any one political party. It is a characteristic—and obvious failing—of politics in democracies where corporate influence is strong and the economic growth ethic forces politicians into a schizophrenic mission—increase growth but decrease the adverse consequences of growth.

The problem appears to be worse in those countries with a greater culture of individualism. Writes one US professor in a nationally syndicated column: 'The government should stay out of personal choices I make. My eating habits or yours don't justify the government's involvement in the kitchen.' The English psychologist Oliver James even differentiates between different capitalist countries in this respect. 'Selfish' (also called 'hard') capitalist economies take a 'look after Number One, bugger everyone else, way of organising things', whereas unselfish (soft) capitalism 'limits personal profits and fosters personal well-being'. According to James, 'the epitome of selfish capitalism is the US, and Denmark is its opposite'. 'Hard' capitalist countries like the US, UK and even Australia, are also those which, according to Dr Richard Wilkinson (referenced in chapter 5), also have the greatest income differentials between upper and lower income earners. Not surprisingly, these countries fare worst on most indices of health, social well-being and crime, than the more 'soft' capitalist countries like Denmark Japan, Norway and Sweden. Little surprise then that European rates of obesity are well below those of the US, which are among the highest in the developed world.

There is a paradox here, however, that needs to be considered before throwing out the politician with the bathwater: even 'selfish capitalist' countries have been highly successful in changing other personal health behaviours. Political scientists Rogan Kersh and James Morone have identified successful government action in four ostensibly similar private areas—drink, drugs, tobacco and sexuality/family planning. Smoking is perhaps the best example, with rates in Australia dropping from a level of around 40 per cent of the adult population who were smokers in the 1970s, to less than 20 per cent today, largely because of strong government action. As pointed out earlier, tobacco, at all levels, is a significant contributor to economic growth. So why the government concern (and success) in reducing smoking, and why can't this be duplicated with obesity?

Following a historical analysis of changes, Kersh and

Morone concluded there are seven triggers to action required to mobilise governments:

1. There must be social disapproval
2. Medical science must have built a body of evidence detailing the harmful effects of the problem
3. Self-help groups should be available
4. There needs to be a demon user (e.g. the type of person that others can dislike)
5. There needs to be a demon industry (e.g. cigarette manufacturers, oil barons), which the public sees as greedily capitalising from the problem
6. There needs to be a mass movement
7. There needs to be interest group action in the issue.

Unlike smoking, not all of these currently apply to obesity. However, according to Kersh and Morone, 'rising social disapprobation, conclusive medical knowledge and further criticism of [the food] industry . . . may fan the flame of interest group activity—including litigation—and result in far more government regulation of fatty foods'.

Meanwhile, what can governments realistically do, not just to reduce obesity, but to capitalise on the developing understanding of the link between obesity and climate change to tackle both obesity (and metaflammation) *and* climate change together?

We will consider three ideas, each designed to have maximal impact on the desired outcome. One is general, one is targeted at increasing physical activity in the community, and one at reducing energy intake. The main aim is to change population attitudes, mainly to over-consumption, but also to the limits of economic and population growth and our responsibility to the ecosphere in a finite world.

In the first place, a Personal Carbon Trading (PCT) scheme as discussed in Chapter 9 would, theoretically at least, support a short-term transition to renewable energy and a modified economic system. Together with some level of corporate carbon limitation aimed at reducing the energy density of processed foods (whether via a tax or a trading system), this should also increase personal energy expenditure and decrease energy intake—the basic requirements for obesity reduction. A PCT system has extra advantage in that, through contraction of purchasable carbon units over time and distribution of units in equal numbers to the whole population, it allows convergence in equality.

Secondly, greater provision needs to be made for low-energy forms of transport by improving public transport, bicycle pathways and pedestrian walkways. Regulation aimed at changing attitudes by allowing greater right of way to pedestrians and cyclists under a wide range of circumstances should also be considered. This is not a hypothetical suggestion, as there are precedents in several European countries. It is not coincidental that as a country develops economically, transport modes shift from walking to bicycles to motorcycles to cars, in line with the rise in obesity (and presumably climate change gases). In 'soft' capitalist countries such as Denmark and the Netherlands, the shift is then back to motorcycles, bicycles and walking. Obesity rates in these countries reflect this.

Thirdly, as pointed out previously, the restriction of high energy-dense (junk) food advertising to children represents the biggest bang for the buck in potential obesity reduction. As this type of food is also highly energy demanding, a reduction in its production would be likely also to have an impact on climate change gases. Governments have typically rejected this suggestion because of pressure from the media and advertising industries that can emphasise their importance—and that of continued consumption—to economic growth. However advertising bans in the UK have been shown to be effective in reducing exposure to children, while having no effect on total advertising revenue. Other possible initiatives include 'traffic light' labelling on foods and fast food outlets (i.e. a green light for those recommended, a red light for those not), and health impact assessments on new food production.

These proposals are suggested to add public health support for personal weight loss programs and prevention initiatives. It was only when such support was given to anti-smoking initiatives (for example, not being able to smoke in public places, advertising restrictions etc.) that inroads began to be made into the smoking epidemic. In doing so, however, we need to know how well current weight loss programs and initiatives work, and what aspects of them can be taken to help one personally reduce or maintain body weight, while also helping to reduce climate change.

What personal initiatives can be taken? In the Monty Python movie *The Meaning of Life*, Michael Palin implores the audience to ponder the meaning of life: '. . . it's nothing very special,' he says. 'Try to be nice to people, avoid eating fat, read a good book every now and then, get some walking in, and try to live in peace and harmony with people of all creeds and nations.' It's taken 100 years of modern scientific research and a bunch of Oxbridge students to come up with what Hippocrates originally proclaimed 2500 years ago as the basis of good health?

The Pythons' take on weight loss might be just as visionary: 'Eat differently and move more!' And they would be no less scientifically correct. Despite the plethora of weight loss programs available, and still to come, that basic principle remains the same.

The public concentration in modern times has been primarily on diets. This is perhaps logical because it is much easier to take 500 calories out of a 3000 calorie per day food intake than it is to add 500 calories of exercise, which would be the equivalent of walking 7 kilometres per day. However, as implied throughout this book, a concentration on weight loss alone, while not recognising the lifestyle risk factors that cause weight gain, is missing the point. It's unlikely even to result in permanent weight loss as it cannot usually be sustained in an environment that encourages and even lauds over-consumption. In any case, all the emphasis on diets appears to have had little impact on the obesity epidemic.

A 2007 review in the US of the published effects of diets found that one-third to two-thirds of dieters regain more weight than they lose on their diets. 'In addition,' the review added, ' the studies do not provide consistent evidence that dieting results in significant health improvements, regardless of weight change. In sum, there is little support for the notion that diets lead to lasting weight loss or health benefits.'

Exercise programs alone are also likely to be less than fully effective in obesity reduction (although possibly of significant health benefit). In pre-industrial societies, sufficient exercise was obtained just staying alive. The reduction in purpose to exercise in modern societies is a reason why organised exercise, such as gyms, workplace programs and so on, is unlikely to fill the gap in required exercise levels to cope with increased food intake.

So how can the relationship between energy intake and expenditure be explained in a way to assist personal weight loss?

In effect this comes down to volume. All effective treatments essentially involve a change in the balance of energy volume, or the amount of calories or kilojoules consumed in relation to those expended. This is shown in Figure 10.1.

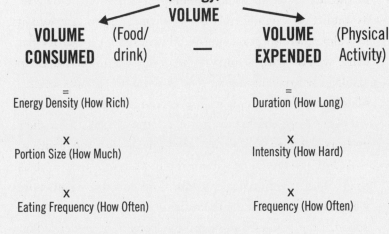

FIGURE 10.1 ENERGY VOLUME AND BODY WEIGHT

Volume (in calorific terms) is defined by three factors on both the input and expenditure side. Although other factors (such as type of nutrient or kind of exercise) may have some independent effects, volume is the key component.

The least understood of these components is probably energy density, on the energy intake side. This is defined as the number of calories or kilojoules per gram of food or millilitre of fluid. Although not yet approved within any guidelines, we suggest an upper cut-off of around 3 calories or 13 kilojoules per gram for food and around 0.4 calories or 1.5 kilojoules for drinks per millilitre. Some foods (eg. nuts) that are higher than that recommended but are quite healthy, should be eaten in small amounts.

On the energy expenditure side, intensity of effort can influence total volume, but as many overweight individuals are also unfit, it is more prudent to increase volume by increasing frequency or duration of effort. It needs to be recognised, too, that the energy balance formula is for weight loss and metabolic health and does not apply to fitness for sporting performance. Yet varying one factor in the equation shown in Figure 10.1 *can* have a significant impact on total volume and hence on body weight.

As with the best picks for public health outlined earlier, we'll now look at three options for achieving personal weight loss, chronic disease prevention and environmental health. Again, one of these is general, one is aimed at increasing personal energy use and one at reducing energy intake.

The general suggestion is to live a low carbon lifestyle, an initiative designed to change our way of thinking about how we live as much as our actual behaviours. Some obvious options for this include growing your own food or buying from local growers' markets, only eating foods with low production and transport costs and using person power rather than machine power whenever possible. Obscure as it may sound, it also means reducing air-conditioning and heating, not so much for the effects on body weight, but on carbon emissions.

The second suggestion related to physical activity, is a psychological one: think of movement as an opportunity, not an inconvenience. This is the first of four physical activity guidelines recommended by the National Health and Medical Research Council in Australia. As a psychological, rather than physical, recommendation, it is intended to change attitudes to the use of personal energy as opposed to machine-related energy. Walking or cycling instead of driving, using stairs instead of lifts or escalators, standing instead of sitting, are all means of recovering the estimated 1000 calories per day lost in the transition from hunter–gatherer to industrialised sedentary worker.

Finally, a shift towards vegetarianism and a reduction in portion size of meals would go a long way to reducing both obesity and the environmental carbon footprint. The reason for a reduction in portion size may be obvious; however, it should be stressed that portions need to also be in the form of low energy-dense foods and drinks. The calorific effects of a reduction in food amount eaten could be easily negated by an increase in the energy density of the food eaten: 200 grams of food averaging 6 calories a gram would have a similar effect on body weight as 600 grams averaging 2 calories per gram (although the effect on greenhouse emissions is less clear).

A shift towards vegetarianism would mean much less energy expenditure in food production, a reduction in gases from animal flatulence and a greater immediate availability of plant-based food sources for humans. The reduced energy density of a plant-based diet would almost certainly also lead to a reduction in population levels of obesity. And although meat-eating is ingrained in modern society, this is closely related to economic growth. Realistically, of course, the world is unlikely to embrace total vegetarianism, for reasons of pleasure as well as economics. However, an increase in this form of eating to, say, two to three days a week at the individual level, would go part of the way to decoupling growth, obesity and the effects on climate change, as well as improving personal health and wellbeing.

The observant reader will note that all of the suggestions made here are contra-indicated by the business-as-usual model of economic growth. And that, of course, is the point. We have suggested that we have passed our sweet spot in economic growth in developed countries. If we haven't, we are likely to be rapidly approaching it. We have also passed the sweet spot in body fat for health and greenhouse gas emissions regulating environmental pollution. Now is the time to seriously look at some of the alternatives to manage these and, in particular, to develop an economic system that more seriously considers human health as well as climate change as dependent variables—before the sweet spots begin to turn sour.

POSTSCRIPT

There is no doubt that the baby boomers (and possibly those born between the two World Wars) in developed countries are among the most privileged human beings ever to have walked upon the face of planet Earth. It's not just that we—for both authors of this book are baby boomers— now live longer (on average) than any previous generation, or that we are the wealthiest generation that has ever lived. It is because we have lived in that tiny window of the most incredibly small percentage of human history and phase of economic development where everything has been right. We've lived through not just one, but at least three sweet spots in human evolution: economic prosperity, good health and a robust environment.

The question that is implied throughout this book, however, is: is it all coming to an end? Have we overshot the sweet spot for economic growth and in doing so increased obesity and chronic disease as well as greenhouse gas emissions associated with climate change? If this is not the case already, is it inevitable that we will overshoot not one, but all three of the sweet spots discussed here in the foreseeable future? Perhaps more disturbingly, will Generation X, those of us who have benefited most from all this, become known as Generation 'X-S' by future generations for squandering our legacy? Have we ignored what the famous twentieth-century ecological economist Nicholas Georgescu-Roegen said when he urged the world, 'not to maximise utility for present generations, but to minimise regret for future ones'?

Industrialised populations generally can't avoid getting fat. It's too late for that. Over two-thirds of industrialised populations (such as the US, Australia and parts of Europe) are overweight or obese. (Japan is a possible exception. Obesity rates here are low in relation to GDP compared with Western countries. It is interesting to note that Japan has a decreasing population, and has significantly reduced growth rates in recent times.) There is more to come, though, with the development of China, India and other emerging countries.

Obesity, however, can be reversed. Indeed, reductions in economic activity have been shown to do this (see Chapter 6). It is less likely that climate change can be reversed as readily.

Of particular concern is the 'boiling frog' effect. This refers to a frog that, when placed in a pot of cold water that is gradually heated, never realises the danger it's in and is boiled alive. It's a common metaphor for disasters that creep up on us a bit at a time. And while the problems of obesity are obvious and (at least superficially) a concern of governments, and climate change is at least attracting worldwide interest, it seems the boiled frog nature of these two problems is nothing compared to getting action on the total economic system. Economists, politicians and financial 'Masters of the Universe' have taken a head-in-the-sand approach to any discussion of modifying the growth system, terrified of the consequences of the alternatives.

Yet if we were to suddenly flick a switch to a non-growth model of economics what would it really look like? We'll leave the next-to-last word to probably the greatest, still-standing exponent of a steady state system of economics, a former member of the World Bank, Dr Herman Daley:

'Simply ask the question: What would the US look like if we had one-half of our current energy consumption? I think there are two ways to kind of get a handle on that. The first is to go back in US history to such a time when we did live off one-half of the current levels of energy consumption. That would put us somewhere around 1960. And gee, life in 1960 wasn't bad. There were all sorts of good things—you were a long way from freezing in the dark, and life was quite good, materially good, and so forth.

'Another way of thinking about it is to take the same year and look for another country with half the energy consumption per capita, like France, and life in France is pretty good. So society could cut energy consumption in half and, if it was done diligently, it wouldn't be a big deal in terms of how it would affect people's welfare. If we limit the scale of the economy, certainly there would be much higher energy costs, and so you just have to make adjustments now toward more efficiency. You would also have to address distribution or equity issues, but these examples show limiting scale doesn't mean wellbeing has to suffer. I believe it could improve.'

Alternatively, we could ask the question the other way round: what would be the consequences of doing nothing? As summed up in the quotation by James Speth at the beginning of Chapter 8: 'All we have to do to destroy the planet's climate and biota [and we could add to this human health] is to keep doing exactly what we are doing today.' It should be obvious that a business-as-usual model is not an option, for either human health and wellbeing or a sustainable environment. Once this fact is appreciated, we can get on with discussing the alternatives—to minimise regret for future generations.

NOTES

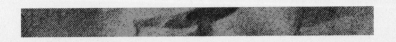

CHAPTER 1 HITTING THE SWEET SPOT

p.3: Albert Einstein see collected quotes from Albert Einstein (http://rescomp.stanford.edu/-cheshire/EisnteinQuotes.html)

p.4: Gaia: James Lovelock initiated the concept of Gaia with his first book, *'Gaia': A New Look at Life on Earth*, Oxford University Press, 1979. Since then he has written several books and over 200 scientific articles on the notion which has come to be accepted as 'Earth System Science'.

p.6: Economic growth: It is important to differentiate between economic growth, as measured in the pure monetary terms of Gross Domestic Product (GDP), and economic development, which can occur through improvements in living conditions, education and other intangibles, often without a financial base.

p.6: Writers warning against unfettered economic growth: These include HE Daly in *Beyond Growth: The Economics of Sustainable Development*. Boston, Beacon Press,

1997; D. Booth in *The Environmental Consequences of Growth: Steady-State Economics as an Alternative to Ecological Decline,* London, Routledge, 1998, and P. Soderbaum *Understanding Sustainability Economics*, London. Earthscan, 2008.

'Collateral damage': Egger G. & Dixon J., 'Should obesity be the main game? Or do we need an environmental makeover to combat the inflammatory and chronic disease epidemics?' *Obesity Reviews* 2009;10 (2):237–49.

'Unintended . . . consequence': Roberts P., *The end of food*, London, Bloomsbury, 2008.

'Inevitable biological response': Oliver J. Eric, *Fat Politics: The Real Story behind America's Obesity Epidemic*, New York, Oxford University Press, 2006.

CHAPTER 2 OBESITY: ITS PART IN OUR DOWNFALL

p.10: Susan Sontag, *Illness as Metaphor*, NY, Picador, 1977.

Percentage of overweight people in developed countries: Australian National Health 2007–08, *Australian Bureau of Statistics*. cat.no 4363.0.55.001.

p.11: Percentage of young people likely to develop Type 2 diabetes: James P.T. et al., The worldwide obesity epidemic. *Obesity Reviews*, 2001;9(Suppl 5):S228–33.

p.11: Percentage of adults likely to develop Type 2 diabetes: AusDiab Study. *Diabesity and Associated Disorders in Australia 2000: The Accelerating Epidemic* International Diabetes Institute, Melbourne, 2000.

'Diseases of modernity': Hodges A.M. et al, 'Modernity and obesity in coastal and highland Papua New Guinea'. *International Journal of Obesity* 1995;19(3):154–61.

p.14: Figures collected by Professor James: See *Obesity Reviews* 2008; 9(Suppl1): *Obesity in China*.

Type 2 diabetes rates in mainland China: Lin L. et al, 'Diabetes, pre-diabetes and associated risks on Minnesota code-indicated major electrocardiogram abnormality among Chinese: a cross-sectional diabetic study in Fujian province, southeast China', *Obesity Reviews* 2009; May 12.

Type 2 diabetes rates in Asia: Juliana C. et al, 'Diabetes in Asia: Epidemiology, Risk Factors, and Pathophysiology', *Journal of the American Medical Association* 2009;301:2129–40.

p.15: A more dynamic formula for body weight: Egger G., Swinburn B., 'An ecological approach to the obesity pandemic'. *British Journal of Medicine* 1997; 315(7106):477–80.

p.17: An often misquoted statistic for obesity: These studies assessed the influence of genes within a very narrow environmental range e.g. within a family or within a single country or culture, thus enormously reducing the measured influence of the environment. Also see Loos R., 'Obesity Facts'. European Conference on Obesity, Amsterdam, March 2009; *PLos Genetics*, 2009, June 5(6): pp 1000508; *Nature Genetics*, 2009; 41(1): 25–34.

CHAPTER 3 GOOD FAT VERSUS BAD FAT

p.19: J.M. Keynes (See www-history.mcs.st-and.ac.uk/Quotations/Keynes.html)

p.19: Obesity throughout history: Bray G., 'Historical framework for the development of ideas about obesity', in Bray G.A., Bouchard C., James W.P.T.(Eds), *Handbook of Obesity*, Marcel Dekker, New York, 1997.

p.21: Vague's findings on body fat storage: Vague J., 'La

differentiation sexuelle: Facteur determinant des forms de l'obésité', *Presse Med* 1947; 55:339–40.

p.21: Scandinavian research confirming Vague's Theories: Wiklund P. et al, 'Abdominal and gynoid fat mass are associated with cardiovascular risk factors in men and women', *Clinical Endocrinology and Metabolism* 2008;93(11):4360–66.

p.22: The role of VAT in disease: Weiss R., 'Fat distribution and storage: how much, where, and how?' *European Journal of Endocrinology* 2007;157:S39–45.

p.22: Obesity-related diseases: Proietto J., 'Obesity and disease: insulin resistance, diabetes, metabolic syndrome and polycystic ovary syndrome', in Kopelman P.G., Caterson I.D., Dietz W.H. (eds), *Clinical Obesity* (2nd ed). Oxford, Blackwell Publishing, 2005.

p.24: Metabolically healthy fat: Taubes G., 'Prosperity's Plague' in *Science* 2009;325:25–260.

p.25: Japanese VAT study: Sasai H. et al, 'Obesity phenotype and intra-abdominal fat responses to regular aerobic exercise', *Diabetes Research and Clinical Practice*, 2009; 84(3):230–8.

p.26: Figure 3.1: Wildman R.P. et al, 'The obese without cardiometabolic risk factor clustering and the normal weight with cardiometabolic risk factor clustering: prevalence and correlates of 2 phenotypes among the US population', (NHANES 1999–2004), *Archives of Internal Medicine*, 2008; 168, 1617–24.

CHAPTER 4 THE ROLE OF INFLAMMATION

p.28: J. Eric Oliver, 'Fat Politics: The real story behind America's obesity epidemic.' Oxford University Press, NY, 2006.

p.28: Hotamisligil's findings: Hotamisligil G.S., Shargill N.S., Piegelman B.M., 'Adipose expression of tumour necrosis factor–alpha: direct role in obesity-linked insulin resistance', *Science* 1993; 259: 87–91; Hotamisligil G., 'Inflammation and metabolic disorders', *Nature* 2006; 444:860–67.

p.29: *The Body at War*: Dwyer J., '*The Body at War* 1988, Allen & Unwin, Sydney.

p.30: Exercise and metaflammation: Pedersen B.K., 'The anti-inflammatory effect of exercise: its role in diabetes and cardiovascular disease control', *Essays in Biochemistry* 2006; 42: 105–17; Woods J.A. et al, 'Exercise, inflammation and innate immunity', *Neurological Clinics*, 2006; 24:585–99.

p.32: Nutrition and inflammation: Egger G., Dixon J., 'Inflammatory effects of nutritional stimuli: Evidence for an evolutionary basis of dietary quality', *Obesity Reviews* 2010;11(2):137–145.

p.33: Table 4.1 and related discussion; Figure 4.1: Egger G., Dixon J., 'Obesity and chronic disease: always offender or often just accomplice?', *British Journal of Nutrition*, 2009; 18:1–5; Egger G. & Dixon J., 'Should obesity be the main game? Or do we need an environmental makeover to combat the inflammatory and chronic disease epidemics? *Obesity Reviews* 2009;10:237–49.

p.33: Zappulla's findings: Zappulla D., 'Environmental stress, erythrocyte dysfunctions, inflammation, and the metabolic syndrome: Adaptations to CO_2 Increases?', *Journal of Cardiometabolic Syndrome*, 2008; 3:30–4.

p.36: Air and bloodstream levels of CO_2: Abolhassani M.,

Guais A., Chaumet-Riffaud P.O., Sasco A.J., Schwartz L., 'Carbon dioxide inhalation causes pulmonary inflammation', *Am J Physiol Lung Cell Mol Physiol*, 2009; 296(4):L657–5.

p.36: Stress and the inflammatory response: Sergio G., 'Exploring the complex relations between inflammation and aging (inflamm-aging): anti-inflamm-aging remodelling of inflamm-aging, from robustness to frailty', *Inflammation Research* 2008; 57: 558–63.

CHAPTER 5 HEALTH, 'ILLTH', ECONOMIC GROWTH AND THE SWEET SPOT

p.41: Francis Delpeuch et al, *Globesity*: A planet out of control. Earthscan, London, 2009.

p.42: A 'schizophrenic response': Sims, LS, *The Politics of Fat: Food and nutrition in America*, New York, Sharpe, 2005.

p.43: US study on health costs of obesity: Reported in the *New York Times*, 28 July 2009.

p.44: US obesity surgery statistics: Robinson M.K., 'The surgical treatment of obesity—weighing the facts', *New England Journal of Medicine* 2009; 361(5):520–21.

p.44: Weighing it Up report: House of Representatives, Standing Committee on Health and Ageing, *Weighing it Up*. Parliament of Australia, 9 May 2009.

p.44: John Ruskin and 'illth': Ruskin J., 'Unto the Last', (1862), in Loyd J. Hubenka (ed), *Four Essays on the First Principles of Political Economy*., Lincoln, University of Nebraska Press, 1967.

p.45: '. . . growth beyond maturity': Bartlett A.A., *Boulder Daily Camera*, 3 Feb, 2008.

p.46: Average longevity: Hopkins E., *Industrialisation and Society: A Social History*, 1830–1951, New York, Rutledge, 2000.

p.46: Decline in infectious diseases: McKeown T., *The Origins of Human Disease*, Basil Blackwell, New York, 1998.

p.47: 'Biggest contributor to human health: Riley J.C., *Rising Life Expectancy: A Global History*, New York, Cambridge University Press, 2001.

p.48: Long- and short-term relationship between growth and health: Tapia Granados J.A., 'Economic growth, business fluctuations and health progress', *International Journal of Epidemiology* 2005;34:1226–33.

p.48: Studies of growth–health relationship: For detailed references of all these studies see Egger G., 'Health "illth" and economic growth: Medicine, the environment and economics at the cross-roads', *American Journal of Preventive Medicine*, 2009, 37(1):78–83.

p.48: University of Michigan study: Tapia Granados J.A., Ionides E.L., 'The reversal of the relation between economic growth and health progress: Sweden in the 19th and 20th centuries', *Journal of Health Economics*, 2008; 27(3):544–63.2007.09.006.

p.48: Health in booms and busts: Tapia Granados J.A., 'Macroeconomic fluctuations and mortality in postwar Japan', *Demography* 2008; 45(2): 323–43.

p.50: 'Tipping point' for climate changes: Intergovernmental Panel on Climate Change. *Climate change: Synthesis Report* 2001. http://www.ipcc.ch/pub/un/syreng/spm.pdf.

p.50: IPAT equation: Sach J., *Common Wealth: Economics for a Crowded Planet*, London, Penguin, 2008.

p.51: Marmot's findings: Marmot M., *The Status Syndrome*, London, Henry Holt & Co., 2004.

p.51: Dr Richard Wilkinson's findings: In Wilkinson R., and Pickett K. The Spirit Level. Penguin, London, 2009.

CHAPTER 6 LINKING OBESITY, CHRONIC DISEASE AND THE ENVIRONMENT

p.52: Edwards P., Roberts I. 'Population adiposity and climate change', *International Journal of Epidemiology* 2009;38(4):1137-40.

p.53: McMichael's research: McMichael A.J. et al, 'Global environmental change and health: impacts, inequalities, and the health sector', *British Medical Journal* 2008; 336(7637):191–94.

p.53: Faergeman's research: Faergeman O., 'Climate change and preventive medicine', *European Journal of Cardiovascular and Preventive Rehabilitation*, 2007; 14:726–29.

New Scientist on economic growth: *New Scientist*, 2008; 2678: 18 October.

p.53: 'The causes of excess weight . . .': UK Department of Health, *Foresight: Tackling obesities—future choices project*, London, Department of Health, 2007. www.foresight.gov.uk/OurWork/ActiveProjects/Obesity/Obesity.asp.

p.54: Figure 6.1: Delpeuch F., et al., *Globesity: A Planet out of Control*, Earthscan, London, 2009.

p.54: Increases in carbon emissions: Trends in Atmospheric Carbon Dioxide—Mauna Loa. Earth System Research Laboratory. Global Monitoring Division. National Oceanic and Atmospheric Administration. http://www.esrl.noaa.gov/gmd/ccgg/trends.

p.55: Global emission statistics: Stern N., *The Economics of Climate Change: the Stern Review*, Cambridge UK, Cambridge University Press, 2007.

p.58: 'I am a planetary physician . . .' Lovelock J., *The Revenge of Gaia*, London, Penguin, 2005.

p.60: Figure 6.2: Egger G., 'Health, "Illth", and Economic Growth Medicine, Environment, and Economics at the Crossroads', *American Journal of Preventive Medicine* 2009; 37(1):78–83.

p.63: 'Degradation of land . . .' Tickell C., 'Foreword' in Lovelock J., *The Revenge of Gaia*, Penguin, London, 2007.

CHAPTER 7 THE PERFECT STORM AND THE SOUR SPOT

p.65: Jeffrey Sachs, *Common Wealth: Economics for a crowded planet. Penguin, London, 2009.*

p.66: Perfect Storm: Junger S., *The Perfect Storm: A True Story of Men against the Sea*, New York. W.W., Norton and Co., 1997.

p.68: Boyle's second decade theory: Boyle N., see http://www.mml.cam.ac.uk/german/news/nbi.pdf. For a report on this see: http://www.abc.net.au/rn/saturdayextra/stories/2009/2544892.htm.

CHAPTER 8 HEALTH PROMOTION FOR ECONOMISTS

p.71: James Gustave Speth. The Bridge at the edge of the world. Yale University Press, New Haven, 2008.

p.73: Steady state economy: Daly H.E., *Beyond Growth*, Beacon Press, Boston, 1996; Daly H. & Farley J., *Ecological economic: Principles and applications*, Washington, Island Press, 2004.

p.72: Growth required under the current economic model: Jackson T., *Prosperity without growth? The transition to a sustainable economy*, Report of the Sustainable Development Commission, March 2009.

p.73: Paradigm shifts in science: Kuhn T.S., *The Structure of Scientific Revolutions*, Chicago & London, University of Chicago Press, 1962.

p.74: 'A stationary condition of capital . . .': Mill J.S., *Principles of Political Economy with some of their Applications to Social Philosophy*, (First published 1848), New York, Prometheus Books, 2004.

p.74: '. . . most of our basic necessities . . .': Oliver J.E., *Fat Politics: The Real Story behind America's Obesity Epidemic*, New York, Oxford University Press, 2006.

p.79: Fall in healthy lifestyles, US: King D.E., Mainous A.G.III, Carnemolla M. & Everett C.I., 'Adherence to healthy lifestyle habits in US adults, 1988–2006, *American Journal of Medicine*, 2009 Jun; 122(6):493–4.

p.79: Rise in obesity, US: Trust for America's Health and the Robert Wood Johnson Foundation, *F is for Fat*, Annual Report, July 2009.

p.80: 'Managers of other people's money . . .': Smith A., *An Inquiry into the Nature and Causes of the Wealth of Nations*, Cannan E. (ed), Modern Library, New York, 1937.

p.82: Sustainable Development Commission quotes: see Jackson T., *Prosperity without Growth* above.

p.82: 'Any water restraint . . .': O'Connor M., *Overloading Australia: How Governments and Media Dither and Deny on Population*, Sydney, Envirobook, 2008.

p.83: 'The politicians will . . . be obliged . . .': Delpeuch F., et al., *Globesity: A Planet out of Control*, Earthscan, London, 2009.

CHAPTER 9 MAKING CORRECTIONS

p.84: Jackson T. Prosperity without growth. Earthscan, London, 2009.

p.85: 'Only a crisis . . .': Friedman M., *Capitalism and Freedom* (40th Anniversary Edition), New York, University of Chicago Press, 1962.

p.86: Organic fuel and greenhouse gases: Intergovernmental Panel on Climate Change, *Climate change: Synthesis Report 2001*, http://www.ipcc.ch/pub/un/syreng/spm.pdf.

p.87: Table 9.1: Fleming D., *Energy and the Common Purpose: Descending the Energy Staircase with Tradable Energy Quotas (TEQs)*, The Lean Economy Connection: London, 2005, http://www.theleaneconomyconnection. net.

p.88: Individual carbon trading, Aubrey Meyer: Global Commons Institute, *Contraction and Convergence: A Global Solution to a Global Problem*, GCI: London, 2006, http:// www.gci.org.uk/contconv/cc.html.

p.89: Air-conditioning and weight gain: Jacobs P., et al., 'The relationship of housing and population health: a 30-year retrospective analysis', *Environmental Health Perspectives* 2009;117(4):579–604).

p.91: Table 9.2: Egger G., 'Dousing our inflammatory environment(s): Is personal carbon trading an option for reducing obesity—and climate change?', *Obesity Reviews* 2008; 9(5): 456–463.

p.92: Deniers' vested interests: Monbiot G., *Heat: How to Stop the Planet Burning*, London, Allen Lane, 2006.

CHAPTER 10 JUST HELP YOURSELF

p.94: The Eagles, 'Long Road out of Eden', Lost Highway records, 2007.

p.96: Longitudinal studies: The Finnish Diabetes Prevention Study (*Diabetes* 2006; 55, 2340–46), the Da Qing study in China (*Lancet* 2008; 371, 1783–89) and the US Prevention on Diabetes Study (*Diabetes* 2005; 54, 1566–72).

p.96: Australian government obesity reports: House of Representatives Standing Committee on Health and Ageing, *Weighing it Up: Obesity in Australia*; Commonwealth of Australia, May 2009, Department of Health and Ageing, Acting on Australia's Weight: A Strategic Plan for the Prevention of Overweight and Obesity, AGP, Canberra, 1997.

p.98: 'Government should stay out . . .?': Quoted in Kersh R.K. & Morone J. (see below).

p.97: James' analysis: James O., *The Selfish Capitalist*, Random House, London, 2008.

p.98: Kersh & Morone analysis: Kersh R., Morone J., 'The politics of obesity: Seven steps to government action', *Health Affairs* 2002; 21(6):14–153.

p.101: UK advertising bans: Office of Communications, 'Changes in the nature and balance of television food advertising to children', 17 December 2008.

p.102: Review of effects of diets: Mann T. et al, 'Medicare's search for effective obesity treatments: Diets are not the answer', *American Psychologist*, 2007; 62(3):220–33.

p.104: Cut-offs for energy intake: Egger G., 'Helping patients lose weight: What works?', *Australian Family Physician* 2008; 37(1/2):20–3.

p.105: NHMRC guidelines: National Health and Medical Research Council, *National Physical Activity Guidelines for Australia*, Australia Government Printing Service, Canberra, 1999.

p.105: Vegetarianism and energy expenditure: Pollan M., *The Omnivore's Dilemma: A Natural History of Four Meals*, New York, Penguin, 2006.

p.105: Vegetarianism and obesity reduction: Kennedy et al., Popular diets: correlation to health, nutrition, and obesity. *Journal of the America Dietetic Association* 2001;101(4):411–20.

POSTSCRIPT

p.108: 'not to maximise utility . . .': Georgescu-Roegen N.,. 'Inequality, limits and growth from a bioeconomic viewpoint', *Review of Social Economy* 1977;35:361–75.

p.108: 'Simply ask the question . . .': Herman Daly interview with ecological economist. Tom Green; CommonDreams. org (31 July 2009).

ACKNOWLEDGMENTS

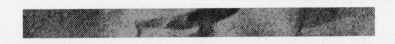

W e wish to thank in particular Dr Tim Gill, Dr John and Sally Padgett, Dr Jose Tapia Granados, Mr Troy Grogan and Dr Ole Faergeman for their comments on the manuscript, and our publisher, Patrick Gallagher, for having the faith to put this to print. Of course they hold no responsibility for the final product. It is to be hoped that we have done them justice in the ideas presented here.

INDEX

Page numbers followed by *fig* indicate figures; those followed by *tab* indicate tables.

adipocytes, 22–23
advertising of junk food,
    100–101
air pollution, 33, 36
alcohol, 31
android body shapes, 21
anti-oxidants, 31, 36

body fat storage
    android and gynoid
        individuals, 21
    ectopic fat, 24
    links to health, 22–27, 26*fig*
    optimum levels, 25
    visceral and subcutaneous
        adipose tissue, 22
Body Mass Index (BMI), 20
body weight. *see also* obesity
    ecological model, 15–18, 18*fig*

energy volume and, 103–104,
    103*fig*

capitalism, hard *versus* soft,
    97–98
carbon emissions, 33–34, 54–55,
    54*fig,* 61–62
carbon trading schemes, 86–90,
    91*tab*
China, 13–14
chronic disease
    effect of lifestyle on, 7, 32*tab,*
        38*tab,* 49–51, 53–54
    global incidence, 13–14
    impact of economic growth
        on, 48–49
    link between obesity and,
        22–23, 29–30, 37–39
    metaflammation and, 29–30

climate change
  as cause of disease, 53–54
  as ecological disturbance,
    58–62
  effect of carbon trading
    schemes, 86–90, 91*tab*
  relationship with obesity,
    52–55
  structural change to counter,
    82–83
climate change deniers, 92
consumption and consumerism,
  8–9, 42–43, 63, 72–73, 75–76,
  78, 81–82, 90, 101
control, 51
corporate behaviour, 79–81, 97
corporate carbon trading (CCT),
  86
counter-argument, 92–93
cycling, 100

decoupling of growth and
  consumption, 72–73
Delpeuch, Francis, 53
diabetes. *see* Type 2 diabetes
diets, 36–37, 102
Dwyer, John, 29

'ecoflammation', 58–59
economic growth
  business-as-usual model, 106
  as cause of obesity, 41, 63–64
  and climate change, 63–64
  drivers, 76
  high consumption and, 42–43,
    75–76, 78, 101
  versus human wellbeing, 6
  negative aspects, 41–42, 45
  population growth and, 76–78

relationship with health,
    45–51, 62–64
ectopic fat stores, 24
Edwards, Phil, 55
election campaign funding,
  79–80
energy density, 104
energy volume, 103, 103*fig*
environment
  effect of personal carbon
    trading on, 91*tab*
  human impact on, 50
epidemiology, 54–57
ethnicity, 22
exercise, 30, 102–103
externalisation of costs by
  corporations, 81
externalities, 81

Faergeman, Ole, 53
fat, 35–36
fat cells
  adipocytes, 23–24
  ectopic fat storage, 24
Flatt, J.P., 15

Gaia, 4–5, 45
global warming, 52–53, 87*tab*.
  see also climate change
government intervention
  against climate change, 82–83
  on obesity, 80, 96–101
  triggers for action, 98–99
Granados, Jose Tapia, 48
greenhouse gas emissions, 33–34,
  54–55, 54*fig*
gross domestic product, 6, 74
gynoid body shapes, 21

health
  economic growth and, 45–51,
    62–64
  effects of personal carbon
    trading on, 91*tab*
healthy food, 31
Hotamisligil, Gokhan, 28–30

'illth', 45, 74
immune system
  and chronic disease, 7
individualism, 97
inflammation
  anti-inflammatory stimuli,
    30–32, 33*tab*
  associated with obesity, 29–30,
    32
  causal stimuli, 30–34, 33*tab*,
    57–62, 60*fig*
  defined, 57–58
  at ecological level, 58–62,
    60*fig*
  nature and role, 29
'inflammatory environment'
  concept, 57

James, Oliver, 97
James, Phillip, 14
junk food advertising, 80,
  100–101

Kersh, Rogan, 98–99

laproscopic gastric banding, 44
life expectancy, 46
lifestyle
  effects on chronic disease, 7,
    32*tab*, 38*fig*, 46–51, 53–54
  low carbon lifestyle, 104–105

vegetarianism, 105–106
  voluntary changes in, 50
limited liability in corporate law,
  80–81
Lovelock, James, 4, 45

Marmot, Michael, 50–51
McMichael, Tony, 53
metaflammation. *see also*
  inflammation
  association with chronic
    disease, 29–30
  association with obesity,
    29–30, 32
  concept, 29–30
  inducers, 30–36
Meyer, Aubrey, 87
Mill, John Stuart, 74
Morone, James, 98–99

Nauru, 46

obesity
  acceptance as health problem,
    19–20
  adipose tissue and, 22
  as cause of chronic disease,
    22–23, 28–29, 37–39
  causes, 14–18
  ecological approach, 15–18,
    18*fig*
  economic impact of, 43–44
  effect of economic growth on,
    41, 63–64
  epidemiological approach,
    7–8
  global incidence, 10–14, 39
  government interventions, 80,
    96–101

inflammatory reaction to, 28–30, 39
population growth and, 78–79
at the population level, 7, 17–18
relationship with climate change, 52–55
obesity prevention measures
effectiveness of government measures, 96–101
need for, 95–96
personal initiatives, 101–106
O'Connor, Mark, 82
O'Dea, Kerin, 47

perfect storms, 65–66. *see also* 'sour spots'
personal carbon trading (PCT), 86–90, 91*tab*
personal control, 51
physical activity
and energy volume, 103–104, 103*fig*
psychological aspect, 105
polyphenol, 36
population growth
and economic growth, 76–78
links with obesity, 78–79

Quetelet, Adolphe, 20
quit smoking campaigns, 92–93, 98

Roberts, Ian, 55
Ruskin, John, 44

SAT (subcutaneous adipose tissue), 22
saturated fat, 35–36

'sick building syndrome', 33
smoking, 36, 92–93, 98
'sour spots'
an approaching global crisis?, 64, 69–70
concept, 66–68
in global history, 68–69
Speth, James Gustave, 79–81
steady state economies, 71–75
stress-related hormones, 36
structural change, 82–83, 85
subcutaneous adipose tissue (SAT), 22
Sustainable Development Commission (SDC), 75, 82, 85–86
sustainable economic growth, 71–76, 82, 85
'sweet spots'
concept, 3–5, 61
in global history, 68–69
overshooting, 5–6
versus 'sour spots', 66–68

tea, 36
transport, low-energy forms, 100
Type 2 diabetes
causes, 11–12
incidence, 11, 14, 23, 46–47
visceral adipose tissue (VAT) and, 22

Vague, Jean, 21
vegetarianism, 105–106
visceral adipose tissue (VAT), 22–23

waist circumference (WC) measure, 21–22

waist-to-hip ratio (WHR), 21–22
walking, 100
weight loss programs
    effect on visceral adipose
        tissue, 25

and energy volume, 103–104,
    103*fig*
Wilkinson, Richard, 51, 98

Zappulla, Donatella, 33–34